Handbook of Sports Medicine and Science

Sports Therapy Services

Organization and Operations

Handbook of Sports Medicine and Science

Sports Therapy Services

Organization and Operations

EDITED BY

James E. Zachazewski, PT, DPT, SCS, ATC

Clinical Director
Department of Physical and Occupational Therapy
Massachusetts General Hospital
Boston, MA;
Adjunct Assistant Clinical Professor
Graduate Programs in Physical Therapy
MGH Institute of Health Professions
Charlestown, MA
USA

David J. Magee, PhD, BPT

Professor
Department of Physical Therapy
Faculty of Rehabilitation Medicine
University of Alberta
Edmonton, AB, Canada

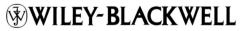

A John Wiley & Sons, Ltd., Publication

Wiley-Blackwell is an imprint of John Wiley & Sons, formed by the merger of Wiley's global Scientific, Technical and Medical business with Blackwell Publishing.

Registered office: John Wiley & Sons, Ltd, The Atrium, Southern Gate, Chichester,
    West Sussex, PO19 8SQ, UK

Editorial offices: 9600 Garsington Road, Oxford, OX4 2DQ, UK
    The Atrium, Southern Gate, Chichester, West Sussex, PO19 8SQ, UK
    111 River Street, Hoboken, NJ 07030-5774, USA

For details of our global editorial offices, for customer services and for information about how to apply for permission to reuse the copyright material in this book please see our website at www.wiley.com/wiley-blackwell

Library of Congress Cataloging-in-Publication Data

Sports therapy / edited by James E. Zachazewski, David J. Magee.
    p. ; cm. – Handbook of sports medicine and science
    Includes bibliographical references and index.
    ISBN 978-1-118-27577-1 (pbk. : alk. paper)
    I. Zachazewski, James E.   II. Magee, David J.   III. International Olympic Committee.   IV. Series: Handbook of sports medicine and science.
    [DNLM: 1. Athletic Injuries–therapy. 2. Athletes. 3. Internationality. 4. Sports Medicine–methods.   QT 261]

    617.1′027–dc23
                                                                2012020850

A catalogue record for this book is available from the British Library.

Cover image: © IOC: Photographers – Field Hockey, Huet; Tennis, Tobler; Ice Hockey, Nagaya; Weight Lifting, Kishimoto; Gymnast, Juilliart
Cover design by Opta Design

Set in 8.75/12pt Stone Serif by Aptara® Inc., New Delhi, India
Printed and bound in Malaysia by Vivar Printing Sdn Bhd

1   2012

Contents

List of Contributors

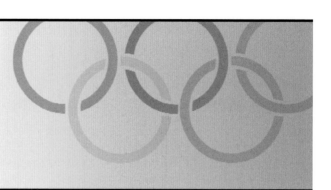

Anderson Aurélio da Silva, MSc
Department of Physical Therapy
School of Physical Education, Physical Therapy &
Occupational Therapy
Universidade Federal De Minas Gerais
Belo Horizonte, MG, Brazil

Caryl Becker, MSc
Chief Physiotherapist
British Olympic Association
London, UK

Natália Franco Netto Bittencourt, MSc
Minas Tenis Clube
Graduate Program in Rehabilitation Sciences
Universidade Federal de Minas Gerais
Belo Horizonte, MG, Brazil

Arthur J. Boland, MD
Department of Orthopaedics
Sports Medicine Service
Massachusetts General Hospital
Boston, MA, USA

Louise Burke, APD, PhD
Head, Sports Nutrition
Australian Institute of Sport
Australian Sports Commission
Bruce, ACT, Australia

Peter Drugge, PT, ATC
Capio Artro Clinic
Stockholm, Sweden

Tommy Eriksson, DN
Stockholms Naprapat Institute AB
Täby, Sweden

Sergio T. Fonseca, PhD
Department of Physical Therapy
School of Physical Education, Physical Therapy &
Occupational Therapy
Universidade Federal De Minas Gerais
Belo Horizonte, MG, Brazil

Randy Goodman, PT, DIP,
Sports PT, BSc
Clinical Specialist in Sports Physiotherapy
University of British Columbia
Kelowna, BC, Canada

James Green II, BS
Graduate Programs in Physical Therapy
MGH Institute of Health Professions
Charlestown, MA, USA

Masaki Katayose, PT, JASA-AT, MSc, PhD
Department of Physical Therapy
School of Health Sciences
Sapporo Medical University
Sapporo, Hokkaido, Japan

Åsa Lönnqvist
Capio Artro Clinic
Stockholm, Sweden

David J. Magee, PhD, BPT
Department of Physical Therapy
Faculty of Rehabilitation Medicine

University of Alberta
Edmonton, AB, Canada

Ron Maughan, PhD
School of Sport, Exercise and Health Sciences
Loughborough University
Loughborough, UK

Luciana De Michelis Mendonça, BSc
INCISA
Graduate Program in Rehabilitation Sciences
Universidade Federal de Minas Gerais
Belo Horizonte, MG, Brazil

Bill Moreau, DC, CSCS
Managing Director, Sports Medicine
United States Olympic Committee
Colorado Springs, CO, USA

Juliana Melo Ocarino, PhD
Department of Physical Therapy
School of Physical Education, Physical Therapy &
Occupational Therapy
Universidade Federal De Minas Gerais
Belo Horizonte, MG, Brazil

Gayle Olson, ATC, MS
Wellness Coordinator
Department of Physical and Occupational Therapy
Massachusetts General Hospital
Boston, MA, USA

Nicola Phillips, PhD, MSc
President, International Federation of Sports
Physical Therapy
Cardiff University
Cardiff, UK

José Roberto Prado Jr, MSc
Centro Universitário Augusto Motta
Rio de Janeiro, RJ, Brazil

Thales Rezende Souza, MSc
Graduate Program in Rehabilitation Sciences
Universidade Federal de Minas Gerais
Belo Horizonte, MG, Brazil

Peter Toohey, ATC, MS
Lake Placid Olympic Training Center
United States Olympic Committee
Lake Placid, NY, USA

Ulrika Tranaeus, DN, MSc
Stockholm Sports Trauma Research Center
Karolinska Institute
Stockholm, Sweden

Tony Ward, M. Sports Physiotherapy
Department of Physical Therapies
Australian Institute of Sport
Belconnen, ACT, Australia

Suzanne Werner, PT, ATC, PhD
Stockholm Sports Trauma Research Centre
Karolinska Institute;
Head of Research
Capio Artro Clinic
Stockholm, Sweden

Lotta Willberg, MD
Orthopedic Surgery
Capio Artro Clinic
Stockholm Sports Trauma Research Center
Karolinska Institute
Stockholm, Sweden

James E. Zachazewski, PT, DPT,
SCS, ATC
Clinical Director
Department of Physical and Occupational Therapy
Massachusetts General Hospital
Boston, MA;
Adjunct Assistant Clinical Professor
Graduate Programs in Physical Therapy
MGH Institute of Health Professions
Charlestown, MA
USA

Foreword

It must be appreciated that a wide variety of professionals are involved with athletes in order to provide these competitors with the highest possible quality of care. In the organization of major sport competitions such as the Olympic Games, careful consideration must be given to the planning and the organization of all services from the immediate medical care to be provided through to the eventual therapies for return to competition.

The co-editors of this handbook, Professor James Zachazewski and Professor David Magee, have assembled a cohort of contributing authors who represent the leading practitioners of the therapies employed with athletes. While earlier publications in the *Handbooks of Sports Medicine and Science* series have dealt with particular sports from the Olympic Summer and Olympic Winter Games and the general topics of sports injuries, sports nutrition, strength training, and sport psychology, this handbook focuses on the pre-event organization, the considerations for international travel, the selection of appropriate therapies, and the specialized roles of specific therapeutic professionals.

A wealth of information is hereby provided for the planning and provision of therapy services for athletes competing in major sport events. We welcome this high-quality addition to the Handbook series!

Dr Jacques Rogge
IOC President

Preface

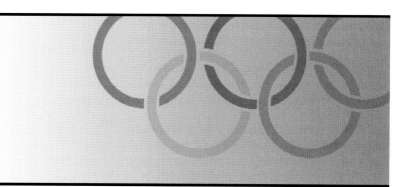

Competitive sports date back to the earliest written recordings of the history of man. The same is also true for the knowledge of sports injuries and their care. The broad collective term used today to describe this body of knowledge and its application to the injured athlete is "sports medicine." While the use of the term "medicine" most often signifies the physicians' contributions to the medical management of the injured athlete, history shows us that much of the care provided to the injured athlete has been rendered not only by physicians but also by a multitude of other professionals. These non-physicians' areas of expertise and concern usually encompass the study and management of the physiological and mental changes and the nutritional requirements as they relate to the injury prevention, the conditioning strategies, and the rehabilitative processes, or the "sports therapies" necessary to prevent injury and return of the athlete to a safe competitive level.

Much has been written over time regarding the "specific therapy" required from a clinical perspective to prevent injury or return of an injured athlete to competition. The editors did not feel that, in a brief publication such as this handbook, we could contribute significantly to this broad body of knowledge. Therefore, our goal in developing this handbook for the IOC Medical Commission was to provide a somewhat unique look at "sports therapy" and contribute a work to the international community that would assist a multidisciplinary professional audience to gain better understanding of "sports therapy" with regard to establishing and delivering the diverse "sports therapy" services required for athletes at international, national, and regional sporting events.

In keeping with the spirit of international cooperation and sharing that the Olympic Games represent, the editors have assembled an international panel of experts and authors from around the globe representing Australia, Brazil, Canada, England, Japan, Sweden, and the United States. Collectively, we have tried to provide the international Olympic community with a guide for the development and delivery of sports therapy services at large international competitions. Each author has not only contributed his or her expertise but, more importantly, also shared his or her practical experience with the reader. In developing the chapters, we have asked the authors to write from the perspective of being a professional consultant hired to provide information regarding sports therapy services in a format that would outline for the reader the issues that must be considered when developing sports therapy services leading up to and during major sporting events.

James E. Zachazewski
David J. Magee

Chapter 1
Sports therapy—Who? What? When? Where? Why? and How?

James E. Zachazewski[1] and David J. Magee[2]

[1]Massachusetts General Hospital, Boston, MA, USA
[2]University of Alberta, Edmonton, AB, Canada

Introduction

When exploring any topic or area of study, one can learn a great deal by asking and answering the questions of Who? What? When? Where? Why? and How?

- What is the definition or meaning of this topic or area?
- Who is this topic or area of study important to? Who is involved in this area?
- When is it important to be aware of this topic and area of study?
- Where is this area of study practiced or important?
- Why is this topic and area of study important?
- How does an individual successfully gain knowledge and competence in this topic and area of study?

Answering these questions allows one to gain overall insight into the topic or area of study and to decide if further exploration is necessary or desired. Included within our answers to these questions are some factors that should be considered in order to develop a strategy to gain further knowledge, competence, and expertise concerning sports therapy.

What is sports therapy?

Sport should be considered in the broadest context when answering the question of "What?" According to the Merriam Webster Dictionary (2010):

> *Sport* is a physical or recreational activity, usually engaged in for pleasure, that an individual is involved in either as a single athlete or participant, or in a group or team format.

As a consequence and requirement of successful sport participation, especially at elite and Olympic levels, various types of training and activities are required. Unfortunately, participation in sport sometimes results in adverse physical or mental/emotional/behavioral consequences to the athlete. Treatment of these adverse physical or mental/emotional consequences often requires some type of *therapeutic* intervention (i.e., the treatment of disease or disorders by remedial agents or methods). The *therapy*, or the treatment of the physical, mental, emotional, or behavioral adverse consequences of sport, is provided by a wide array of professionals to allow the athlete to return to practice and/or competition. The definition, number, type, background, educational preparation, expertise, and experience of these health care professionals vary broadly on an international basis. This variability may be due to history, culture, sport bias, economics, or access to therapeutic resources to name but a few. In many countries, Olympic committees and professional associations have established minimum requirements for clinicians who wish to work at Olympic events or facilities. For the purpose of this book, the term "sports therapy" is best defined as "the provision of non-surgical, non-pharmacologic interventions by a broad array of professionals to help the athlete alleviate the adverse physical, mental, emotional or behavioral adverse consequences of sport and allow the athlete to return to an optimal level of health, well being and competitive function."

Who practices sports therapy

There are a multitude of professionals who support an elite athlete from a clinical therapeutic basis. The type of therapy delivered, and which professional will provide that therapy, may differ from country to country. This difference in delivery may be based on things such as educational preparation, licensure requirements (if any), availability, and the cultural environment of the country and sport. In many cases, there is overlap of what individuals in each profession may provide relative to another professional. Some of the types of overlap that may exist are summarized in Table 1.1 (Booker and Thibodeau 1985).

That being said, one must never forget the importance of the "psychological bonding" between the athlete and the health care professional. This bonding can lead to increased confidence and comfort of the athlete when dealing with different health care professionals.

Sports Physiotherapist. Physiotherapy (or *physical therapy* as termed in the United States) is defined as "the treatment of disease, injury, or disability by physical and mechanical means (using massage, regulated exercise, water, light, heat, and electricity)." Depending upon the country, physiotherapy was established as a profession soon

after the end of World War I. As a result, physiotherapists have played a significant role in the therapeutic management of injured Olympic and Para Olympic athletes almost since the inception of the modern games. The establishment of the role and skill set of the physiotherapist through the utilization of exercise, massage, and other therapeutic means goes back much earlier, to the time of the ancient Greeks and Romans, as can be seen when reading Chapter 2, "A History of Sports Medicine and Sports Therapy." Modern day "sports physiotherapists" also play a prominent role in the emergency management of injuries that may occur during competition or training. The education, training, and professional preparation of physiotherapists vary from country to country. The general course of study and initial preparation of physiotherapists has great breadth, taking into consideration all ages, and types of pathologies, diseases, and injuries. In all instances, sports physiotherapy is a further course of study and area of subspecialization, after initial generalist preparation, and commonly, these physiotherapists have specialty certification in sports therapy to deal with the unique requirements and care of athletes. This system of training allows for greater breadth and depth of preparation combined with specific topics applicable to sport, and the care and prevention of sports injuries by the sports physiotherapist. Education and training to become a sports physiotherapist vary from country to country with educational preparation ranging from different types of certification to bachelors, masters, and clinical doctoral degrees. Training of physiotherapists generally and specifically for sports physiotherapy tends to follow a medical model in most countries. Many sports physiotherapists, when not directly involved with sports teams, work in hospitals and private clinics.

Athletic Trainer. Athletic training is a profession and course of study that is found predominantly in the United States, although some other countries such as Canada and Japan have also seen the development of this profession. The role that the athletic trainer plays with the Olympic level athlete may be similar to that of the sports physiotherapist depending upon the sport and country. The education and preparation of the athletic trainer centers around athletic-, sport-, and

Table 1.1 Functions of the sports therapist

Prevention	Assessment	Treatment and Management
Preparticipation examination • Medical history • Physical examination • Profiling Proper conditioning Protective equipment • Selection • Fitting • Maintenance Safety supervision • Facilities • Equipment Preventive techniques • Taping • Padding • Bandaging • Braces Observing athletes • Recognize problems and minor injuries Hygiene • Rest • Diet Assessment techniques • Recognize injury • Determine severity of injury • Determine when athlete can return to activity Emergency care procedures • Supplies • Plane of action • Immediate care Rehabilitation strategies • Prevent reinjuries • Strengthen previously injured area Monitoring environmental conditions Range of motion (flexibility) Muscular strength and endurance Coordinated movements Functional activities Cardiovascular endurance Assessment techniques • Evaluation of effects of rehabilitation program	Emergency assessment Primary survey • Airway • Breathing • Circulation Secondary survey • History • Observation • Palpation • Stress tests Evaluation of findings • Medical referral • Treatment application Maintain records • Injuries • Treatment Facilities • Inspection • Safety • Sanitation Equipment and supplies • Purchasing • Maintaining Health care services • Organize • Communication • Policies and procedures Emergency support services	Immediate first aid • Ice • Compression • Elevation • Rest Follow-up treatment • Therapeutic modalities • Exercise programs Protective techniques • Taping • Splinting • Padding • Supporting • Immobilizing Assessment techniques • Evaluation of the effects of treatment procedures on signs and symptoms Previous injuries and present status • Medical history • Requirements of each Health topics • Knowledge of health education Social and personal problems • Knowledge of available professionals • Knowledge of situation requiring consultation • Referral procedures Knowledge of team or family physician Instructing student trainers Continuing education

Adapted from Booker and Thibodeau (1985).

activity-related injuries and conditions, with significantly less preparation across the age, pathology, and disease spectrum than the physiotherapist receives in their entry level generalist education/preparation. Overall, there is a greater depth of preparation at the entry level relative to athletic injuries and their management. Educational emphasis is placed on sport mechanics, injury prevention, emergency management, and therapeutic intervention across a wide variety of sports. Educational preparation is at the bachelors or masters degree level. Training of the athletic trainer has historically followed a kinesiology/physical education and physical activity model. However, many programs in the United States are beginning to evolve in schools of allied health with curricula that match credentialing requirements. Most athletic trainers (or athletic therapists as they are called in Canada), when not involved full time with sports teams, work in educational institutions (high schools, colleges, and universities) or along with sports physiotherapists in private clinics.

The role of the athletic trainer and sports physiotherapist are often similar and may have significant overlap when it comes to treating athletes. A generic term "sports therapist" is used to indicate both a sports physiotherapist and/or an athletic trainer. Some of the functions of these individuals are shown in Table 1.1. The utilization of athletic trainers versus sports physiotherapists varies based on sport, country, and culture. Overlap of knowledge, skills, and abilities can foster maximal efficiency and expertise being directed at the care of the athlete as well as controversy, competition, and "turf battles." The most effective professionals of either profession will tend to foster an area of trust, mutual respect, and sharing of expertise regardless of their background to work to the advantage of the injured athlete.

Coach/Trainer. The coach (or trainer, as called in some countries) of an athlete is the individual who trains an athlete or a team to compete through instruction in sporting techniques and skills, designing season plans, and teaching safe and effective practices. They act as the planner and organizer, providing motivation and mentorship for individual athletes and individuals on teams. This individual, working with others, is the person the athlete most commonly identifies with and works with to achieve his or her maximum potential to compete. Depending on the country, these individuals may have gone through a specific training program, often with different levels of certification or may have gained their knowledge by being involved in sport. Those who are trained in specific programs commonly come from a

kinesiology/physical education and physical activity model.

Massage Therapist. Massage has been used as a therapeutic method of treating the injured athlete since the earliest reported history of sport. It is perhaps the most common "therapy" provided across the many countries who participate in the Olympics. The professional education, background, and training of the massage therapist/masseur vary greatly from country to country. In some countries, specific educational preparation, course work, examination, and licensure are required, while in others, apprenticeship and mentoring under a master or acknowledged expert is the common method of preparation. Guided and graded experience, success with the athletes treated, and acceptance by the athlete and team are common requirements of all massage practitioners. Techniques and methods may vary from country to country and from practitioner to practitioner; however, the purpose is the same. Massage is used before, during, and after events to prepare the athlete for peak performance, to help them recover following competition or practice, or as part of injury treatment (to prevent injury from occurring).

Strength and Conditioning Coach. Professionals with specific expertise in the areas of strength training and conditioning participate with almost all teams. The main area of responsibility for these coaches/therapists is to assure the appropriate level of sport-specific conditioning for the athletes allowing them to obtain peak performance at the time of the games. While often termed "coaches," the strength and conditioning coaches are of expertise and responsibility often times overlap with those of various other "therapists" (e.g., physiotherapists and athletic trainers) depending on where the athlete is in terms of preparation, injury, rehabilitation, recovery, or conditioning. Communication is paramount between everyone working together to allow the elite athlete to attain world-class performance and results. The educational level and preparation of coaches/trainer again varies depending upon the country and the culture of a particular sport. Preparation can range from college and graduate/doctoral level course work, examination and licensure to apprenticeship, and mentoring under a master or acknowledged expert in that particular sport or activity.

Sports Psychologist. Obviously, one of the key factors in success in any sport or athletic event is the level of physical function of the athlete (i.e., strength, speed, endurance, agility, flexibility, and balance to name but a few). However, the emotional and psychological factors associated with sport and success require just as much attention, although this is often underrecognized and underappreciated. For this reason, the sports psychologist is a critical member of the sports therapy team. The educational preparation, background, and training of this professional allow them to concentrate and address the nonphysical needs of the elite athlete at a critical junction in their career. Such an individual deals with the emotional health of the athlete and can assist them in visualizing success and optimal performance of a skill required "to medal," conquering issues of confidence and fear, coping with an injury should it occur, burnout and depression, or coping with poor performance should such an event occur. While all members of the therapy team must have an appreciation for the emotional and psychological well-being of the athlete at the time of competition, the skills that the sports psychologist brings to the therapy team are critical. They have the depth and resource that others may not have.

Chiropractor. Chiropractors are often asked to work as part of a collaborative multidisciplinary health care team. In this setting, their clinical duties, like most sport therapists, are focused primarily on diagnosis and management of musculoskeletal conditions. Once a diagnosis is made, common treatment techniques employed by the chiropractor include joint manipulation and mobilization, soft tissue manipulation, rehabilitative exercise, taping, bracing, and nutritional and lifestyle modification. Many of these skills may overlap with other sport therapists, especially the sports physiotherapist and/or athletic trainer. Athletes often seek the manual therapy skills of the chiropractor during competition, and this has resulted in increased demand in chiropractors.

In the United States, it is important to distinguish chiropractors with specialty certification in sport from the unspecialized chiropractic physician. Chiropractors certified by the American Chiropractic Board of Sports Physicians (ACBSP) have additional training in diagnosis and management of sports injury, concussion, emergency procedures, taping and bracing, and preparticipation examination. Most chiropractors come from a science background and when not involved with sports teams, work in their own private practices.

What makes a good sports therapist (characteristics and commitment of a sports therapist)?

Attitude and Dedication. As a group, sports therapists, regardless of whether or not they are a physiotherapist, athletic trainer, or chiropractor; massage therapist; strength and conditioning coach; sports psychologist; or some other type of health care professionals demonstrate great passion not only for their chosen profession but also for their dedication to the sport and the athletes who entrust them with their care. Overall, the sports therapist should demonstrate a positive, "can do" attitude at all times to the athlete and the team. A sports therapist needs to make sure that the athlete knows that he or she is there for the athlete when the athlete needs him or her the most—at time of injury and/or adversity. Sports therapists should display a quiet but recognized air of confidence in their own skills and abilities, their ability to assist the athlete overcome physical and emotional adversity, at what may be the most critical time of the athlete's career. The sports therapist must demonstrate the ability to remain calm, focused, and able to help in the most stressful situation.

Training and Knowledge Base. Any sports therapist associated with a sport must have a high level of skill, knowledge, ability, and expertise in their chosen profession that is recognized by their peers and the athletes/teams with whom they work. The sports therapist must not only have knowledge of injuries and the management of injury and illness associated with the sport from a "clinical" perspective but he or she must also have a thorough understanding of the specific skills and techniques required within a sport. This knowledge allows the sport therapist to have insight into the correct biomechanics and pathomechanics associated with the sport and with injuries and illness that may result from participation. The sports therapist must also respect and gain insight and knowledge into the culture, psychosocial components, attitude, and values of the participants and coaches involved in the sport. When injury and/or illness occur, all of these components are intimately woven together and must be managed for a successful outcome.

Flexibility and Time Commitment. Any sports therapist knows that flexibility is a key component for success with a sport, team, or elite athlete. The sport therapist must be willing to flex his or her schedule to accommodate to changes in practices and event schedules. These changes often occur at the last minute and often need accommodation. Because of this, as well as the time required for such things as travel and meetings, the time commitment required for a sports therapist involved in sports is significant. Depending on the sport and the time within the sports season, practices may be at various times of the day or night. Travel is often required. This travel may take the sport therapist away from his or her home for up to weeks or months at a time. These time commitments have an impact not only on the sport therapist's professional and personal life, but they may have a significant impact on the lives of their families as well. While the rewards from being associated with an elite team or group of athletes provide great satisfaction, the time spent away from home can have an adverse impact on family.

When and where is the sports therapist needed?

Sports therapy is needed by the athlete not only during his or her competitive season/event but also during the off-season/training season. The type and amount of therapy service needed by the athlete will vary by sport and season. Access to competent, highly trained sports therapists is needed not only at central training sites but also where individual athletes and teams may train when not at an identified central training site.

During the competitive season, athletes need to access sport therapy services throughout their active training cycle often on an acute, urgent basis. The urgent need and access to intervention is meant to allow the athlete to minimize injury and illness that occurs while still allowing the athlete to vigorously train and compete. Intervention provided is often times aggressive in nature, based on the short window of the competitive season. Intervention strategies are aimed at allowing the injured athlete to continue to participate despite the injury and to minimize the progression of the injury if possible. Therapy services are provided not only within the clinical setting but also at the venue/practice/competition site. When an athlete or team is traveling, the therapist must often be creative in determining where the "clinic" will be to treat the injured athlete. Hotel rooms, buses, or an open area of the venue/arena often must become the therapists' clinical office.

During the noncompetitive training season, access to sports therapy services may vary greatly depending on the athlete, sport, country, culture, and sophistication of the organization or governing body of the sport. During this noncompetitive, training season, athletes are often away and geographically distant from centralized sophisticated therapy services available to them during the competitive season. It is in this situation that great care must be taken by the individual athlete and organization to find the best possible therapy resource available in the athletes' geographic area. This is often difficult to do. Efforts should be made by the governing body to attempt to develop a network of therapists willing and able to provide the athlete with any necessary therapy services in the geographic area that a particular athlete or team is staying during the noncompetitive training season.

Why is sports therapy important?

The "sports therapist," regardless of their area of clinical expertise, is a critical member of the sports medicine health care team for any athlete. Often, it is the sports therapist with whom the injured

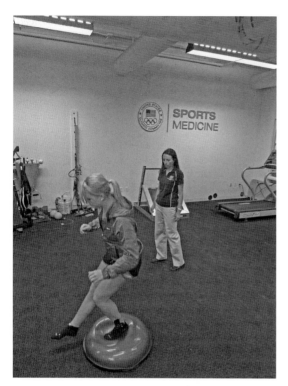

Figure 1.1 Supervision and oversight of a functional rehabilitation exercise by sports therapist

athlete interacts with the most during the acute management of their injury, rehabilitation, recovery, and ultimate return to competitive status (Figure 1.1). The therapist and athlete often develop a strong bond of trust and confidence based on a shared goal of expeditious return to activity and success.

How does one become a sports therapist?

Acquiring the knowledge, skills, and abilities to work as a sports therapist with the elite athletes of the world requires time and dedication to one's profession. Most often, the acquisition of training and knowledge about a particular sport or group of athletes is gained through multiple mechanisms:

• *By having been an athlete in that sport before becoming a sport therapist.* Many former athletes go into various health care professions and return to work with sports in which they previously participated. This real-world experience not only gives them significant insight into the sport from a technique and skill perspective but also allows them to understand how an injury or illness could affect an individual athlete, coach, or team from a "cultural" and value perspective.

• *By gaining experience and insight from working with a specific sport or specific types of athletes over a number of years.* Experience in this manner helps the sport therapist develop a significant knowledge base, even if he or she has not personally participated in the sport.

• *By having a mentor.* "Master" sport therapists, recognized and acknowledged by their peers, athletes, and coaches, often identify new, young staff with great potential to work with athletes. After identification, the mentor progressively facilitates and guides the development of his or her protégé/apprentice within a sport community. This mentorship and guided experience allow the "master" sport therapist to pass on his or her knowledge and expertise while assuring optimal care for the team and athletes associated with a particular sport. The process of mentorship can be developed formally in conjunction with academic preparation (such as the completion of identified fellowships or residencies that meet specific criteria established through professional association's or country's National Olympic Committee or a specific sports' national governing body) or informally through specific sports or with sport therapists already involved with teams.

• *By completing appropriate course work and academic preparation.* Academic preparation ranges from initial "entry" level education to various advanced degrees and types of subspecialization, often involving many years of study and examination. This academic preparation allows the sport therapist to understand and utilize the most current methods and techniques of clinical care available. Academic preparation may also include postgraduate/licensure residencies and fellowships that meet specific preidentified criteria for some type of accreditation. Academic or clinical preparation should be "evidence based" to the greatest extent possible. However, the sport therapist must recognize the impact that culture, tradition, and coaches/athletes stating "this is how we have always done it" have on a sport. A sport therapist, no matter how knowledgeable, who does not recognize or cannot work within a sport's existing culture or tradition will not be successful. Although it may be needed for optimal care, change must respect existing values of a sport and work through experiential success to effect change. Academic preparation must be combined with experience and understanding of the specific needs of sports and athletes for optimal preparation and efficacy of practice.

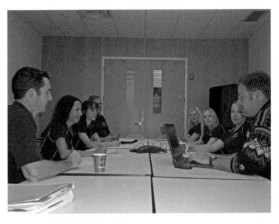

Figure 1.2 Multidisciplinary group meeting to discuss status of the needs of injured athletes that the group is working with for efficient effective return to competition

Summary

"Sports therapy" is made up of many different professionals all with the common goal of assuring the health and well-being of the elite Olympic athlete so that the athlete may compete at the highest level possible. The professionals have unique and overlapping knowledge, skills, and abilities. The collaboration and creation of a "team" of professionals will provide the athlete with the best sports therapy approach to support them in their quest for athletic excellence and success (Figure 1.2).

References

Booker, J.M. & Thibodeau, G.A. (1985) *Athletic Injury Assessment*. CV Mosby Co., Toronto.
Merriam Webster's Dictionary (2010). Springfield, MA.

Chapter 2
A history of sports medicine and sports therapy

James E. Zachazewski[1], Arthur J. Boland[1], and Nicola Phillips[2]

[1]Massachusetts General Hospital, Boston, MA, USA
[2]Cardiff University, Cardiff, UK

Introduction

Sport and athletics date back to the earliest written recordings of man's history (Figure 2.1) as does the knowledge of athletic injuries and their care. Writings describing sports injury date back to the book of Genesis 32, and writings describing the use of exercise in a therapeutic manner in the provision of health care for an injured athlete date back to the writings of the Hindus and Chinese around 1000 BC. Throughout the ages, our knowledge and ability to prevent, diagnose, and care for athletic injury and illness have continued to progress. With progress, multiple disciplines of professionals have developed specific bodies of knowledge and expertise aimed at improving our ability to prevent and provide the most appropriate care for the injured athlete. "Sports medicine" is the broad collective term that we utilize today to describe the body of knowledge and application of this knowledge to the injured athlete. While the use of the term "medicine" most often signifies the physicians' contribution, history will show us that much of the care provided to the injured athlete has been rendered not only by physicians but also by a multitude of other professionals.

Defining "sports medicine" and "sports therapy"

Using Merriam-Webster Dictionary as a foundation, "sports medicine" may be best defined as the art and science dealing with the maintenance of health and the prevention, alleviation, or cure of disease or injury in the athlete. It includes the study of the management of musculoskeletal injuries and the medical problems encountered by athletes during training and competition and training. Sports medicine also encompasses the study of the physiological and mental change and nutritional requirements placed upon individuals involved in strenuous athletic activity, injury prevention and conditioning strategies, and the rehabilitative process, or "sports therapies" necessary to prevent injury and return athletes to a safe competitive level. "Sports therapy" may be best defined as the art and science of the application of remedial agents or methods to prevent injury and return an injured or ill athlete back to a state of optimal physical condition to return to sport. "Sports medicine" and "sports therapy" incorporate the expertise of exercise physiologists, nutritionists, physical therapists, athletic trainers, massage therapists, chiropractors, strength

Sports Therapy Services, First Edition. Edited by James E. Zachazewski and David J. Magee.
© 2012 International Olympic Committee. Published 2012 by John Wiley & Sons, Ltd.

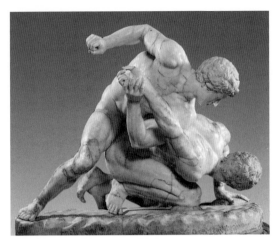

Figure 2.1 Wrestling from ancient Greek games (*Florence, Galleria degli Uffizi*) (Reproduced from Koursi (2003))

and conditioning coaches, and sports psychologists, as well as a team of physicians and surgeons (Figure 2.2). These are indeed specialties and disciplines that have made significant contributions to our understanding and management of sports-related injuries throughout history.

Because of the obvious overlap in the knowledge and expertise of many of these groups of professionals throughout the remainder of this chapter, we will use the term "sports medicine" to

collectively describe the contributions of all professionals dedicated to the health and well-being of athletes entrusted to their care.

Where and when did sports medicine and sports therapy begin?

Recreation, entertainment, competition, exercise, dance, and athletic activity have been part of man's history since the dawn of time. As far back as 2500 BC, drawings have been discovered in Egypt in the tomb of Beni-Hassan depicting exercise, ball games, lifting, wrestling, and physical competitions (Figure 2.3). As recorded history continues so does man's desire for athletics and competition. Frescos dating to the Minoan civilization of 2000 BC depict boxing, wrestling, and bull jumping. Athletics and competition do not occur without injury. Although no records are available regarding specific injuries, we know that some must have occurred and we can only assume that someone knowledgeable in the management of these sport-related injuries provided care for the injured athlete.

The first recorded athletic competition, which was described by Homer in the Iliad, consisted of athletic events subsequently included in the ancient Olympic Games. These games were the Funeral Games for Patroclus, organized by his friend

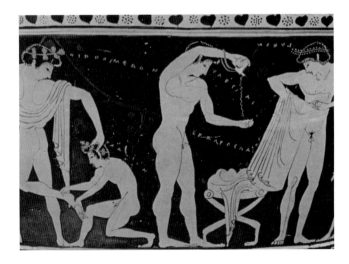

Figure 2.2 Depiction of ancient Greeks pre-game preparation with assistance of physicians and trainers (*Red-figure krater by Euphronions, ca. 510 B.C. Berlin, Staatliche Museen*) (Reproduced with permission from Art Resource New York, NY, USA)

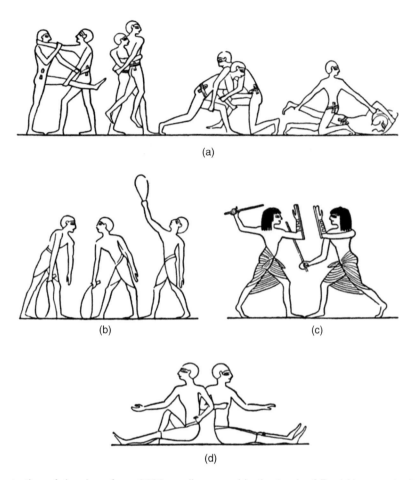

Figure 2.3 Illustration of drawings from 2500 BC discovered in the tomb of Beni-Hassen depicting exercise, ball games, lifting, wrestling and other physical competitions (*Beni-Hassan, l.c.*) (Reproduced from Gardiner & Litt (1987) with permission from Ares Publishers, Chicago, IL, USA)

Achilles. In the Iliad, Homer also identifies two physicians Machoan, a surgeon, and Podalirius, a physician, who accompanied the Greek troops to Troy (Figure 2.4). Effective in treating injured soldiers, and even performing surgical procedures, one can only assume that these experienced physicians may have also been available to treat the injuries incurred by athletes involved in the Funeral Games, given the importance that the Greeks placed on sport. Based on those assumptions and the breath of sports medicine, perhaps Machoan and Podalirius were not only the first "games doctors" but also the first sports physiotherapists and athletic trainers.

Ancient times

It has been stated that Herodicus, who lived in the 5th century BC, has been stated to be the father of sports medicine. Although his writings no longer exist, his medical contributions and reputation have been documented by his contemporaries, Hippocrates, Plato, and Aristotle, as well as by Galen in the 2nd century AD and the authors of the earliest textbooks of medical history. What best qualifies Herodicus as the father of sports medicine is that, prior to entering medicine, he was educated

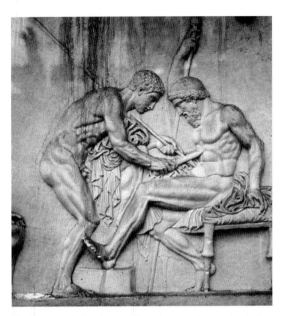

Figure 2.4 Ancient Greek carving depicting Machaon and Podalirius described in the Iliad by Homer (*A Roman bas-relief at Herculaneum National Museum, Naples*) (Reproduced from Margotta (1967))

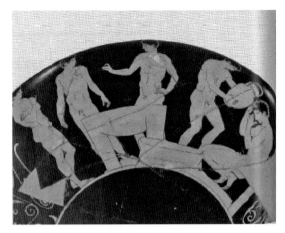

Figure 2.5 Recovery after exercise in ancient Greece. Young men washing themselves after exercise. In the gymnasia a special area called the Loutron was set aside for the young athletes to cleanse their bodies and refresh themselves after exercise (*London, British Museum*) (Reproduced from Koursi (2003))

and worked as an athletic trainer. Traditionally, during the 5th century BC in Greece, physicians were not allowed into the gymnasia where the athletes were practicing and conditioning under the supervision of trainers. Herodicus, however, had a close association with the athletes as a sports trainer and during that time had the opportunity to establish a treatment philosophy centered on the importance of diet and exercise as it related to health and disease (Figure 2.5).

In the western world, the use of the term "therapeutic exercise" is first associated with Herodicus in the 5th century BC. Herodicus used "aggressive rehabilitation" in his treatment programs, recommending both stringent diets consisting of primarily grains and strenuous exercise, especially prolonged walking. The techniques and treatment protocols used by Herodicus were not without criticism, however, due to their excessive physical demands. In fact, his contemporaries, including Hippocrates, Plato, and Aristotle, criticized some of his programs as being potentially harmful to some patients. Although Plato stated that Herodicus "belonged, no doubt, to the rank of fully accomplished physicians," and that he applied the "principles of gymnastics to the treatment of disease and the preservation of health," some of the treatment protocols used by Herodicus were excessive. Seven hundred years later in the 2nd century AD, Claudus Galen of Rome, who may perhaps be called the first "team physician," would term the theories and treatment protocols of Herodicus harsh and potentially injurious.

By the 5th century BC, the "trainer-coach" had developed into a significant force in Greek athletics, even forming guilds with requirements for membership. The "trainer" was expected to be an expert on massage, diet, physical therapy/conditioning, and hygiene, as well as coaching in the areas of boxing, wrestling, jumping, and other sports. Although not a "physician," the "trainer" played a significant role in the health and well-being of the athlete, assuming many roles specifically provided by a multitude of specialty providers today (e.g., athletic trainer, massage therapist, nutritionist, sports physical therapist). One of the most famous trainers was Milo of Croton. One of Milo's training

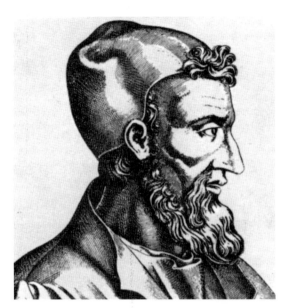

Figure 2.6 Graphic of Galen, the first "team physician" (*Sixteenth-century engraving. Bertarelli Collection, Milan*) (Reproduced from Margotta (1967))

methods to gain strength was to start lifting a bull on the day of its birth, and doing so daily thereafter so that one could lift the animal when it was full grown—providing us with the first record of a progressive resistive exercise training program.

Unfortunately, close collegial practice did not exist between physicians and trainers early in the first millennium due to professional jealousies. Physicians did not participate in the care and training of the athlete except to treat the injuries until about the 2nd century AD. The insight, presence, and the naming of Claudius Galen of Pergamum and Rome as physician to the gladiators would change this. Galen is the first team physician (Figure 2.6).

Galen was born in 131 AD in Pergamum in Asia Minor where he was appointed the physician at the gladiator school by Pontifex Maximus. He was subsequently brought to Rome by the Emperor Marcus Aurelius to provide care for his own family as well as the gladiators and athletes. During his career, he carried out well-documented studies in exercise physiology and reported upon the effects that training, exercise, and nutrition had on individuals of

all ages. As a teacher and scholar, his contributions included not only medical works but treatises in philosophy, grammar, mathematics, and law.

Galen was very much in favor of athletic activities, pointing out in his treatise on the small ball, and how light, as well as progressively more challenging exercises, could have beneficial effects on the bodies of all age groups, including children and the elderly. However, he condemned the professionalism and excessive practices that were increasingly evident among the competitive Olympic athletes. The abuses he commonly observed among the professional and Olympic athletes of his day had begun during the ancient Greek period. These abuses may also parallel some of the problems we continue to encounter today. He deplored the specialization of athletes, particularly boxers and wrestlers, which rendered their bodies overweight and out of proportion to the point where they were unfit to participate in other sports or military duty. He noted that many of these athletes subsequently developed significant disabling medical problems after their competitive years, which often led to premature death. Although there is evidence that the ancient Babylonians, Assyrians, Egyptians, Chinese, and Indian civilizations participated in athletic activities and undoubtedly had medical practitioners who may have functioned as team physicians and sports medicine doctors before the time of the Roman Empire, Galen's verifiable scientific contributions and impressive body of writings justify the label that Dr. George Snook gave him as "The Father of Modern Sports Medicine."

After Galen, throughout the first millennium and well into the second, the progression of medical knowledge was somewhat stifled with the rise of mediaeval church. Despite this, however, there is evidence of discussion and description of the value of exercise in the prevention and treatment of injury. In the 5th century, Aurelianus described the use of weights and pulleys as an effective form of exercise. He recommended their use, along with hydrotherapy, even for postoperative rehabilitation.

The scientific heritage of the Greeks and Romans was preserved and saved from destruction by the Byzantine Empire and Islamic culture in the Middle East. The Father of Muslim medicine, Hakim ibn-e-Sina (or Avicenna as he is known in the West) living in the 10th century summarized what was known up to that time by compiling the medical writings of the ancients. Many of the writings promoted the use of medical gymnastics, massage, and warm baths to promote rehabilitation. In the 11th century, Maimonides from Egypt also wrote extensively about the value of therapeutic exercise taken in moderation.

As the second millennia progressed in the 15th century, Vittorino de Feltre and Maffeuseginus introduced obligatory exercise into educational curricula. A six volume textbook set on "The Art of Gymnastics" by Gerolamo Mercuriale was a pivotal contribution, purchased and utilized by both the public and medical professions. In these books, Mercuriale classified exercise into preventive and therapeutic categories (Figure 2.7). These texts remained in print for more than 150 years. The utilization of exercise was championed further in the 16th century by Joubert who introduced therapeutic exercise in medical school curricula and Pare (the great barber surgeon) who was the first to point out that exercise was indispensible in the recovery of function after the primary treatment of fractures. In the early 17th century, in 1602, Marsilius Cagnatus of Verona published a book entitled "Preservation of Health" in which he encouraged physicians who had knowledge of sports to become more involved in the supervision of athletic contests. Cagnatus recognized how important it was for the physician to have an interest in and an appreciation of the demands of the various sports in order to provide effective care. A critical observation and fact that remains true today.

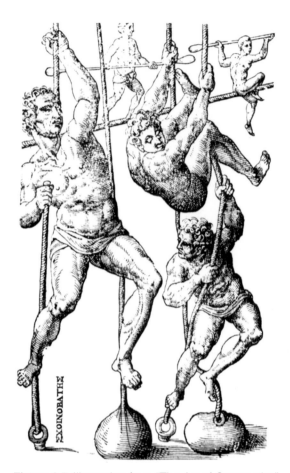

Figure 2.7 Illustration from "The Art of Gymnastics" by Geroloamo Mercuriale from the late 1500's depicting therapeutic exercise using rope climbing (*Mercurialis, Hieronymi: De artis gymnastica, libri sex, ed. 4. Venice, Iuntas, 1601*) (Reproduced from Peltier L.F. (1985), with permission from Lippincott Williams & Wilkins)

Modern times—organizational development

The term "sports medicine" had its origin at the beginning of the 20th century in Europe. "Hygiene in Sports" was a two volume set published in 1910 by Seigried Weissbein of Berlin that described the injuries encountered in athletes and outlined various treatment options. Weissbein's work was followed in 1914 by a chapter on sports injuries in the "Encyclopedia of Surgery" by G. Van Saar. The first sports medicine society, The German Society for Sports Medicine and Prevention, was formed in Germany in 1912. Unfortunately, the outbreak of World War I interfered with the interest and concern physicians had with sports injuries.

Since the beginning of the 20th century, sports medicine has developed as an area of special interest and expertise at an accelerating pace. National and international organizations and societies have developed to allow members from across the globe to share expertise, information, research, and experience to better care for injured athletes. It would be impossible in this short chapter to present information on all of these invaluable organizations. We have chosen a few to highlight and provide examples of professional societies that foster the growth and development of the area of sports medicine.

International Federation of Sports Medicine (FIMS). With the return of the modern Olympic Games, international interest was rekindled in sports medicine. In 1928 at the Second Winter Olympics in St Moritz, Drs. Kroll of Switzerland, Buytendijk of Holland, and Latarjet of France met with 33 other physicians and planned the First International Congress of Sports Medicine that was held at the 1928 Summer Olympic Games in Amsterdam. A total of 280 sports physicians from 20 countries attended the first congress. The organization formed was originally known as the Association International Medico-Sportive (AIMS), but in 1933 was changed to Federation International Medico-Sportive et Scientifique, FIMS. FIMS is an international federation of the national sports medicine organizations of more than 100 countries around the world. FIMS continues to hold regular scientific meetings, has representatives and participating members from around the world, and makes significant contributions to the science and specialty of sports medicine. Since the origin of FIMS, many nations have established their own national sports medicine organizations and have collaborated in regional and international educational and scientific programs.

American College of Sports Medicine (ACSM). As noted previously, Europeans had established an international sports medicine organization, FIMS, well before the need for one was recognized in North America. Following World War II, the sports medicine physicians in the United States recognized the value of a collaborative effort and founded the American College of Sports Medicine in 1954. The multidisciplinary membership of the ACSM consists of a broad spectrum of clinicians (physicians, surgeons, physical therapists, athletic trainers, etc.) and scientists (basic and applied science, exercise physiology, etc.) interested in sports medicine who continue to meet regularly and publish their findings in their journal, *Medicine and Science in Sport, Exercise and Sports Science Reviews, Health and Fitness Journal,* and *Current Sports Medicine Reports.* This remains a highly respected and productive organization that addresses the full spectrum of sports medicine issues within the United States and the international community.

International Federation of Sports Physical Therapy. The International Federation of Sports Physical Therapy (IFSPT) is a worldwide Federation, which is a recognized subgroup of the World Confederation of Physical Therapy (WCPT) and was established by sport specialty subgroups of National Physiotherapy Professional Organizations across the world. The IFSPT was developed in 2000 and currently has 24 national member organizations. The intention of IFSPT is to be the international resource for sports physical therapists to promote their profession through professional medical organizations. IFSPT has compiled internationally recognized competencies in sports physiotherapy and this document is the basis of the criteria for recognizing specialist practice in this specialist group of the profession. Some member countries, such as the United States, United Kingdom, Australia, Holland, Denmark, Ireland, and New Zealand, already have established professional development pathways toward specialist status. Each country has developed a pathway that reflects their cultural and professional environment. However, the IFSPT Registration Board has developed an assessment process that acknowledges national differences while establishing parity of standards for specialist status. IFSPT specialty recognition is also possible through individual application in countries postgraduate specialist education, although some countries are now working toward doctoral level for specialty recognition.

Sports Physical Therapy Section. The Sports Physical Therapy Section (SPTS) of the American Physical Therapy Association (APTA) is an example of one of the national organizations comprising membership of IFSPT. SPTS was established in 1973 by 75 physical therapists dedicated to a career in sports physical therapy. Specialty status within SPTS is achieved through board certification examinations, in conjunction with the American Board of Physical Therapies Specialties (ABPTS) and was initially established in 1986. As of 2011, there are a total of 824 sports clinical specialists (SCS). In contrast to this assessment process, other IFSPT member country sports physiotherapy specialty organizations, such as Sports Physiotherapy Australia and the Association of Chartered Physiotherapists in Sports Medicine (UK), use a combination of portfolio-based submission and Masters level assessment in various forms. The *Sports Physical Therapy Sections* journal, *The Journal of Orthopedics and Sports Physical Therapy*, which was begun in 1979, is currently the largest physical therapy publication with a circulation of more than 6600.

World Federation of Athletic Training and Therapy. The World Federation of Athletic Training and Therapy (WFATT) is a multidisciplinary organization of national professional bodies representing health care practitioners who manage and rehabilitate injuries in sport and physical activity. Members of this organization represent various professional groups such as athletic trainers, physiotherapists, sports rehabilitation therapists, and sports therapists. Membership is wide ranging and more than one health care practitioner group from any country can become a member of WFATT.

National Athletic Trainers Association. The National Athletic Trainers Association (NATA) is a professional organization within the United States and is a founder member of WFATT. NATA members work collaboratively with team physicians providing services for athletes ranging from immediate/emergency injury management; injury prevention; preseason, in-season, off-season conditioning programs; and rehabilitation/return to play programs. In 1971, a certification examination was introduced to assure the competence of the graduates of the athletic training programs, which has a minimum of BSc level preregistration education. This organization has continued to evolve and grow since its inception in the 1950s, assuring the growth of the profession and contributing significantly to the body of knowledge we term "sports medicine." By 2008, there were 352 accredited college programs in North America and the membership in NATA had grown to more than 30,0000, attesting to the interest in and significance of this as a career. In Canada, a similar organization (the Canadian Athletic Therapists Association) has evolved following a similar pathway. The NATA publishes a well-respected journal, *The Journal of Athletic Training*.

Based on the history we have presented earlier in this chapter, it would appear that the profession known as athletic training in the United States extends back to the early Greeks and Romans. Other countries have differing titles for this role, such as sports trainer, sports rehabilitation therapist, while in other countries, the role is considered a postregistration specialty within physiotherapy, as opposed to a separate profession.

International Society of Arthroscopy, Knee Surgery and Orthopedic Sports Medicine. The International Society of Arthroscopy, Knee Surgery and Orthopedic Sports Medicine (ISAKOS) was formed in 1995 and held its first meeting in 1997. ISAKOS was developed from the merging of two other professional associations—the International Society for the Knee (IKS), which was formed in 1977, and the International Arthroscopy Association (IAA), which was founded in 1974. This organization has grown significantly with the addition of international members from numerous countries and all continents. Membership is open to individuals, rather than member countries around the world. Along with FIMS, ISAKOS has become an important and respected international sports medicine society.

American Orthopaedic Society for Sports Medicine. The American Orthopaedic Society for Sports Medicine (AOSSM), created in 1972, evolved from the American Academy of Orthopaedic Surgeon's Committee on Sports Medicine, which was founded in 1964. The founding members of the AOSSM recognized the need for an orthopedic subspecialty society dedicated to sports medicine, which would provide a more effective vehicle for collaborative studies, research, and educational programs. During the years since the AOSSM, the parent Academy of Orthopaedic Surgeons has passed the responsibility and leadership in providing sports medicine educational programs for its members to the AOSSM. In 2008, there were more than 2000 active members in the AOSSM. The research and educational materials submitted and presented at its meetings have been published in the *American Journal of Sports Medicine* since 1972. Members of the AOSSM have established certified orthopedic sports medicine fellowships within their academic and clinical practices, and following completion of one of these accredited fellowships, the fellows can take the formal certification examination to become credentialed as a sports medicine specialist.

American Medical Society of Sports Medicine. The American Medical Society of Sports Medicine (AMSSM) was formed in 1991 and held their first meeting in 1992. The AMSSM was originally conceived and developed by internists and primary care sports medicine physicians, emergency medicine, and family or internal medicine physicians who saw the value of forming their own primary care subspecialty organization. Most of these founding members were also members of the American College of Sports Medicine or had done sports medicine fellowships with their orthopedic colleagues. The membership had grown to more than 2000 members by 2010. Members of the AMSSM produce excellent research and clinical studies that are printed in their publication, the *Clinical Journal of Sports Medicine*. The AMSSM also collaborates to produce the annual team physician's courses that are cosponsored with the AOSSM and the ACSM. Members of the AMSSM are able to take a certification examination that qualifies them as credentialed sports medicine specialists. A similar organization in Canada is called the Canadian Academy of Sport Medicine.

Summary

Sports medicine is an ancient medical subspecialty whose roots stretch over two centuries and has attracted the interest, scientific talent, and enthusiasm of many medical practitioners and scientists throughout history. The interest of individuals in athletic activity and the unfortunate results created by injury and illness require a broad array of professionals with the knowledge, skills, and expertise necessary to render the best care possible. This need is answered by the sports medicine practitioner, whether he or she is a physician, therapist, trainer, masseur, nutritionist, psychologist, or other.

In addition to the national and international organizations mentioned earlier, individuals and organizations have produced important basic science and clinical studies on sport-specific as well as anatomic region-specific injuries. Time and space does not allow one to mention all of the important contributions that have been made throughout history or to list all of the impressive surgical and rehabilitative advances made which have allowed athletes to more quickly and safely return to competition. It is clear that the problems created by sports injuries are of global interest, and therefore, it is important that clinical and scientific cooperation continue both internationally and regionally so that further advances in our understanding and management of athletic injuries may occur.

An historical review of sports medicine is by necessity selective, and therefore may be criticized as being incomplete. Many books have been written about the history of medicine from ancient civilizations up to the present time, incorporating the achievements of physicians from many continents and numerous societies. We sincerely apologize to those individuals and organizations whose contributions we have failed to include in this chapter.

Recommended readings

Allbutt, C. (1921) *Greek Medicine in Rome.* McMillan & Co., New York.

Appleboom, T., Rouffin, C. & Feirens, E. (1988) Sport and medicine in ancient Greece. *American Journal of Sports Medicine*, 16, 594–596.

Aristotle, Rhetoric, 1.5.1361b5.

Boland, A. (2011) History of sports medicine. In: L. Micheli (ed), *Encyclopedia of Sports Medicine*, pp. 664–672. Sage Publications, Los Angeles, CA.

Darling, E. (1899) The effects of raining, a study of the Harvard University Crew. *Boston Medical and Surgical Journal*, CXLI, 205–221, 229–233.

Galen, On the Therapeutic Method 1.1.6.

Galen, iii.31, vol. Xviii p. 88.

Gardiner, E.N. & Litt, D. (eds) (1987) *Athletics of the Ancient World*, p. 90. Ares Publishers, Inc., Chicago, IL.

Garrison, F. (1929) *History of Medicine*, 4th edn. W. B. Saunders Co., Philadelphia, PA.

Georgoulis, A., Kiapidou I., Velogianni L. *et al.* (2007) Herodicus, the father of sports medicine. *Knee Surgery, Sports Traumatology, Arthroscopy*, 15, 315–318.

Hippocrates. De Morbis Vulgaris. Vi3 Vol. iii, p. 599.

Hippocrates. Epidemics 6.3.18.

Hitchcock, E. (1885) Athletics in American colleges. *Journal of Social Sciences*, 27–44.

Jackson, D. (1984) The history of sports medicine, part 2. *American Journal of Sports Medicine*, 12, 255–257.

Jokl, E. (1980) Pioneers, professor A.V. Hill, a personal tribute. *Journal of Sports Medicine*, 20, 465–468.

Jouanna, J. (1999) *Hippocrates*, pp. 3–55. Johns Hopkins University Press, Baltimore, MD.

Koursi, M. (ed.) (2003) *The Olympic Games in Ancient Greece: Ancient Olympia and The Olympic Games*. Ekdotike Athenon S.A., Athens.

Margotta, R. (1967) *The Story of Medicine* (edited by P. Lewis). Arnoldo Mondadori Editore, Milan.

Nichols, E. (1906) The physical aspect of American football. *Boston Medical and Surgical Journal*, CLIV, 1–8.

Nichols, E. (1909) Football Injuries of the Harvard squad for 3 years under revised rules. *Boston Medical and Surgical Journal*, CLX, 33–37.

Peltier, L.F. (1985) *The Classic: Geronimo Mercuriali (1530–1606) and the First Illustrated Book on Sports Medicine*. Lippincott Williams & Wilkins, Philadelphia.

Peltier, L. (1987) The lineage of sports medicine. *Clinical Orthopaedics and Related Research*, 216, 4–12.

Plato, De Rep. Lii. p. 406.

Plato, Phaedrus. 227d.

Plato, PROTAG. 20. p. 316.

Ryan, A. (1978) Sports medicine history. *The Physician and Sports Medicine*, 77–82.

Ryan, A. (1974) *Sport Medicine*, pp. 3–29. Academic Press–Elsevier Science Technology, Maryland.

Snook, G. (1978) The Father of sports medicine. *American Journal of Sports Medicine*, 6, 128–131.

Snook, G. (1984) The history of sports medicine, Part 1. *American Journal of Sports Medicine*, 12, 252–254.

Soranus, Vita Hippocrates, 2.175,77 lib.

Chapter 3
The role and importance of the sports therapist: pre-event, event, and post-event

Suzanne Werner[1,2], *Peter Drugge*[2], *Tommy Eriksson*[3], *Åsa Lönnqvist*[2], *Ulrika Tranaeus*[1], *and Lotta Willberg*[1,2]

[1]Karolinska Institute, Stockholm, Sweden
[2]Capio Artro Clinic, Stockholm, Sweden
[3]Stockholms Naprapat Institute AB, Täby, Sweden

Introduction

The Olympic Games is not solely an adventure of 16 days but considerably longer. The preparations for an Olympic Games event start some 2–3 years before the opening of the games. This means that the medical teams of the different national sports federations and the National Olympic Committee start a long-term planning process with the goal of having all athletes healthy at the start of the Olympic Games and maintaining their health throughout the games. While athletes play the central role at the Olympic Games, they must be appropriately supported by their coaches and medical team. Therefore, the most important issues for the medical team are to see that the athletes are healthy at the start of the games and stay healthy throughout the games.

The athlete's perspective

An elite athlete at the Olympic level expects and appreciates being supported and treated by a sports therapist with high level of skill and knowledge about both rehabilitation and the athlete's specific sport. The sports therapist's knowledge about the sport should include knowledge of the rules of the sport, especially as they apply to the care and treatment of injuries during the competition, as well as technical and tactical factors involved in the sport. This knowledge helps the sports therapist gain the athlete's trust and confidence relative to the impact an injury or illness may have on the athlete's ability to compete, and to work effectively with the athlete to develop an appropriate strategy and plan to maintain the ability to compete should an injury or illness occur. A sports therapist who has been active as an athlete himself or herself has the advantage of understanding what the athlete is going through during training and competition, when health is affected and/or an injury occurs. This experience is highly appreciated by most athletes as it allows the therapist and athlete to develop a relationship of trust and confidence.

An elite athlete expects to be treated immediately when he or she has sustained an injury and should be able to start the treatment and rehabilitation as soon as possible (Figure 3.1). Athletes feel that every hour and day that treatment and rehabilitation are delayed can be decisive. Delays in care can adversely affect an optimal outcome and return to normal sports performance in the shortest time possible. Expeditious care involves not only that provided by

Sports Therapy Services, First Edition. Edited by James E. Zachazewski and David J. Magee.
© 2012 International Olympic Committee. Published 2012 by John Wiley & Sons, Ltd.

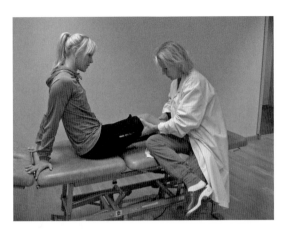

Figure 3.1 Physician examining an injured soccer player

the sports therapist but all members of the sports medicine team.

The treatment should be geared toward the functional return of the athlete to his or her sport and therefore should be individualized for each athlete (Figure 3.2). Physical examinations should be performed regularly throughout the entire rehabilitation period in order to develop the best possible gradual increase of sports-specific training. Communication between the sports therapist and the athlete and coaches is essential. The sports therapist must work closely with the coaches and other

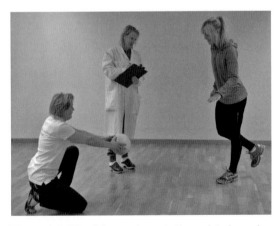

Figure 3.2 Physician and sports therapist observing injured soccer player. Treatment should be geared toward the functional return of the athlete to her sport

trainers involved with the athlete to plan the most appropriate return of the athlete to his or her sport without adversely affecting their condition, injury, or illness. The sports therapist should discuss the athlete's injury with the athlete and coach explaining the injury, healing times, and how long it will take to return to the sport and to competition. This ensures everyone is "on the same page" with regard to the athlete's care and is extremely important for a safe return to sport avoiding new injuries or a reinjury.

Following his or her return to sport and activity, the elite athlete may need help with planning and carrying out injury prevention exercises not only to return to optimal sports performance but also to attempt to minimize the chance of recurrence. Athletes who have confidence in a particular sports therapist and his (her) knowledge, skill, and expertise in maintaining the athletes' health and condition often develop a bond of mutual trust, respect, and confidence. Contact is maintained over time often resulting in a relationship that lasts not only during the athlete's competitive days but throughout life.

Chief medical officer's (CMO) perspective

Forming a medical team

Prior to the Olympic Games, it is important to build a medical team consisting primarily of physicians and sports therapists. The team should meet prior to the games to discuss working strategies to ensure optimal care for the athletes. The whole medical team is at the games to serve all of the athletes (and often support staff) at the games regardless of the type or size of the sport. There should be at least one physician and one sports therapist in the team's medical center in the village at all times. While musculoskeletal problems or injuries and other trauma are the most common issues dealt with by the sports therapist, the medical team may have to deal with other medical issues as well (e.g., influenza, doping issues). Therefore, it is important to have sports medicine physicians and orthopedic sports surgeons represented on the medical team.

The Olympic Village

It is important that each member of the medical team is aware of all the medically related services that are offered by the host country in the Olympic Village. Sports therapists should know where practice and competition sites are relative to the Olympic Village. The chief sports therapist should contact the CMO, or preferably the chief sports therapist, of the organizing committee to get information about how the medical facilities will be organized and what equipment they will have in the village. It is important that each country's National Olympic Committee understands the importance of having one or two single rooms not occupied in case someone needs to be placed in quarantine during the games. Furthermore, in each country's medical team area, there should be some rooms for physical therapy treatments, and one secure room for the physicians where the door can be closed and locked for storage of pharmaceuticals and medical equipment.

Prior to leaving his or her country for the Olympic Games, the sports therapist should look closely at the competition schedule and determine the level of activity (i.e., the number of events and location) for each day so that a preliminary plan can be developed for positioning of the medical team during these days. The sports therapist should be aware of weather conditions expected at the times of the games. This is especially true if there is a risk for hot and humid weather to ensure proper care of the team's athletes under these conditions (e.g., appropriate fluids and electrolytes).

At the games, the medical team should meet every evening after the competitions for that day have been completed and debrief going over the happenings of the day and outlining any issues that have arisen during the day. If another sports therapist is going to "take over" for a particular colleague the next day, this also provides an opportunity to bring the new sports therapist up to date on any issues involving the athletes and team and to work out the next days schedule together. Issues

such as which sports and athletes will be competing the next day, any special needs from any athlete or coach, any athlete or team needing support during training, and any injured athletes needing treatment and/or support can be discussed. Every member of the medical team should have a written schedule of what he or she will be doing the next day.

The physician's perspective

To serve as a physician at an Olympic Games means that the physician has become one of the leaders of the medical team for that country. Depending on the country and the size of the team, the physician may be the CMO for that team or one of several physicians involved with the team. If the physician is the CMO, he or she will be the leader of the medical team and will be responsible for the planning of each physician's schedule (and in some cases, the sports therapist's schedule) and making decisions about injury risks and illnesses, and issues related to doping. Furthermore, the CMO and other physicians support the sports therapists. The CMO debriefs the medical team and administrative staff in cases of really severe injuries related to the team or if something goes wrong (e.g., doping issues). Each member of the medical team has the responsibility to keep a high working morale and good spirits within the medical team. To be a physician at an Olympic Games means that forgetting your "normal role" as a physician sometimes becomes mandatory, especially during the event. Physicians should expect to be involved in activities other than those that are typical for his or her profession, or specialty practice area. It may not solely be to treat a medical (or perhaps mental) problem of an athlete but also to make sure that everything that is needed at the competing sports arena is available when needed. Furthermore, the physician may also be needed as a support for the sports therapist when deciding the treatment of an acute injury. Another important issue for the physician is to be able to effectively communicate and explain to the injured athlete and his or her coach about different possible treatments should injury or illness occur and their impact on the athlete's ability to continue to compete. Thus, a physician is part of a team and when not occupied with his or her professional duties, he or she helps where needed with other more general tasks.

Preparation of equipment

A great deal of the medical team's work and preparation should be done before the start of the games (usually at least 1 year in advance of the games). Lists of what equipment and supplies that the medical team should bring to the games will need to be made. This will make it easier to avoid forgetting anything that might be needed during the games, and it will also make it easier when filling out the necessary forms for customs on entry to the host country. Sponsors are often sought for surgical equipment, supplies, and medications in order to keep costs as low as possible. Equipment and supplies left over from previous games should be inspected and repaired where necessary and out-of-date supplies discarded. Commonly, items being shipped leave your country some months prior to the opening of the village. Therefore, it is necessary to start to plan and execute early. The CMO should develop a close working relationship with the head sports therapist—as the need for mutual support and help will be more than either can imagine.

Health screening

It is crucial that each country's National Olympic Committee allows mandatory screening of all athletes' health prior to the games. Both physicians and sports therapists should play an active role in reviewing the health reports of their Olympic athletes. Medications of the athletes should be reviewed to ensure there are no doping issues and that the team will have ample supplies of the drugs needed by the athletes. The medical team should be aware of and review "the doping red list" and the doping classifications and approved medications that are not banned for competition. Every effort should be made to make sure that if an athlete is taking a banned substance for a medical condition that the appropriate waiver has been received from

the IOC prior to the competition. The medical team should make sure they have a copy of any wavers.

Team physicians will also treat all members of the country's team for medical issues including the administrative staff in case of injury or illness during the games. Therefore, health declarations should be received from each member of the team and administrative staff prior to the games. Support personnel often are older and often have different spectra of illness, injury, or diseases than the athletes.

The athlete's confidence in the physician

It is important that the physician and sports therapist who will be working with specific teams and/or athletes get to know each individual athlete in order to establish good rapport and confidence that might be needed during the games if difficult medical decisions have to be made. Understanding the rules will prevent a physician or sports therapist from doing something wrong during the competition that could cause the athlete to be disqualified. In order to become familiar with the sport, the medical team should study the literature and watch competitions. The more one knows about the specific sport, the better he or she will be able to establish trust and confidence with the athlete and coach, which will make medical treatments easier. Each medical team member should bring his or her medical kit or bag as it will make one feel safe and "at home" during the games.

Ideally, the medical team should arrive at the Olympic Village before the games start. This will make it easier for the medical team to have a chance of getting acquainted with the athletes and coaches as well as the transportation system and practice and competition sites. At least one member of the medical team should meet and talk to the athletes and their coaches in order to find out their needs and to discuss how the medical team can support them during the games and their specific competitions. At least one physician and one sports therapist should be in the medical room at the village all the time during the games.

The medical team members should become familiar with the village and what it offers as well as the host country's general medical facility or "village hospital." At this early stage, one can set up the medical area for the team in the assigned area, visit practice and competition sites to see what the medical set up is at these venues, and check where the doping control will take place.

Once the games begin, medical team members should report to each other during the day if there are any changes from the schedule that was decided the night before. All medical team members should support each other throughout the entire games, keep up good spirits, mood, and be positive! The medical team and facilities and the atmosphere projected there are essential for the well-being of the athletes.

When the games are over, the athletes and medical staff should be allowed to evaluate the medical service and staff, offering both positive and negative criticism. It is only through evaluation that the service can be improved.

The Olympic therapist's perspective

Preparations before the Olympic Games

In Sweden, the members of a preliminary medical team are chosen approximately 10 months before the games. The number of medical team members depend both on how many athletes qualified for the games and their coaches. About 10 months prior to the Olympic Games, the whole national team including the athletes, the coaches, and the medical staff are brought together at an "Olympic Camp." Here, the athletes receive a lot of information (e.g., about the city where the Olympic Games are held, the venues, transportation, the Olympic Village, and the organization around the national team). Team members are fitted for their Olympic clothing and informed about different team buildings and competitions. The medical team is gathered together for a careful planning of equipment, the distribution of the work, working conditions, and discussions about things such as scheduling and doping.

It is a great advantage if the medical team has the possibility of visiting the Olympic Village before the event to become familiar with the rooms of the clinic, the equipment to be used, and transportation to different venues. Furthermore, it is valuable for the medical team to be able to meet with the organization committee in order to receive information about what the medical services will be offered and about the doping controls and visit any hospitals that may be used during the Olympic Games.

Sports therapists attending the Olympic Games need to be current about the latest treatment methods especially for sports-specific problems and injuries. They also need to be familiar with more uncommon injuries and their treatment in order not to jeopardize an athlete's sports participation if he or she sustains a more rare injury. If an athlete comes to a sports therapist with an injury that he or she is not familiar with, the sports therapist should ask his or her colleagues about what to do rather than "try" a treatment that may be wrong and thereby threaten sports participation. Furthermore, it is not unusual that "Quick-fix" treatments are sometimes used, but they should not result in future health problems for the athlete.

It is also important to initiate collaboration with the sports therapists from the different federations in order to collect further knowledge and competence and thereby improve and reinforce the competence of the whole medical team. The goal is to provide each athlete with the best possible treatment. In order for collaboration to work optimally, the following factors are extremely important: treatment principles and sharing the parts and areas of responsibility. Sports therapists commonly work alone in their own sports federation and making their own decisions. However, at the Olympic Games, it is of utmost importance to have good collaboration with other sports therapists in order to give the injured athlete the best possible treatment.

Prior to the Olympic Games, each country has its own methods of preparation. It is very good if it is possible to arrange a pre-camp in the right time zone and the same climate as where the Olympic Games will take place. Time difference means that an acclimatization of about 24 hours is needed for each hour of time difference. Furthermore, 7–10 days are needed to become acclimatized to heat.

The time prior to the start of the Olympic Games is another area that needs attention and careful preparation by the medical team. Issues such as keeping the athletes as healthy as possible, prevention strategies to be used, support during the training sessions, competition and rehabilitation when injured must be discussed and solutions found prior to the games.

Equipment

In order to fully prepare the athlete for physical performance and to treat his or her symptoms and injuries at the Olympic Games, a variety of equipment is needed, such as equipment for electrotherapy, different rehabilitation tools, as well as different types of bandage and tape and other materials.

24-hour service during the Olympic Games

The medical team will serve both the athletes and their coaches and support staff whenever needed each day and night at the Olympic Games. Every evening when the athletes and their coaches are back from the practice and competition sites, the medical team should meet to discuss what has happened during the day and to make plans regarding the different tasks for the next day. Each sports therapist is responsible for the athletes of his or her own sport. However, the sports therapist needs to be prepared to work with athletes and their coaches in other sports due to many injured athletes in one sport, a sport not having a dedicated sports therapist, or an athlete having a special injury in a sport that is not the sports therapist's own sport.

In the Olympic Village, the host country also has a "polyclinic" that is open 24 hours a day with selected times (e.g., 7 AM to 8 PM service) for specialties including a dentist. Radiological examinations, ultrasound, and magnetic resonance imaging (MRI) are also commonly available in the Olympic Village "polyclinic." The "polyclinic" also has a physical therapy clinic with sports therapists who mainly treat athletes from small nations that have no medical support of their own.

Traveling with teams—Is the therapist just "a therapist"?

Other roles of the therapists

To travel with athletes at a national level provides a fantastic experience but often also requires long days of hard work. It means high levels of stress and the need and ability to come to rapid decisions. The acute treatment following an injury and the immediate start of the rehabilitation are a small part of a great number of tasks performed by the sports therapist. Injury prevention is something the sports therapist works for continuously. This is very important before the Olympic Games as well as during the event. In addition to injury prevention strategies and treating injuries, the sports therapist often takes care of other needs that the athlete has (e.g., personality and/or psychological issues). Some athletes need time just for a talk. This may not necessarily be due to an injury but the specific situation such as not knowing whether he or she will be chosen to play the match today or not, which can lead to frustration and stress on the part of the athlete. Often the sports therapist will be the one who has a chat with this particular athlete in order to offer him or her support and encouragement. Therefore, the sports therapist at an Olympic Games needs to be aware of and prepared for all kinds of different tasks. Working at an Olympic Games as a sports therapist is a rich and rewarding experience that will provide fantastic and unforgettable memories that will enrich one's life!

Chapter 4
Hosting international Olympic events: providing host therapy services at major games

Randy Goodman

University of British Columbia, Kelowna, BC, Canada

Introduction

One of the most rewarding challenges therapists can have in their career is playing host to the visiting medical teams at various major games. The author had the privilege of "welcoming the world" to Vancouver, Canada, for the 2010 Winter Olympic and Paralympic Games. While the concept of being a manager of therapy services for any "games" is daunting, if one is an organized person with lots of energy, the rewards can be outstanding.

In this chapter, the whole "host" concept, from the planning stages through transfer of knowledge once the games have concluded, will be explored. Each concept will be looked at from various viewpoints including venues, athlete villages, services for countries or teams who do not have therapy personnel, and assistance to those countries who do have therapy personnel.

The most important concept is to comprehend what hosting actually means. According to Webster's Dictionary (2011), a host is defined as "one who receives or entertains guests socially, commercially, or officially; one that provides facilities for an event or function." One of the reasons for our great success hosting the world's therapists at the 2010 Winter Games in Vancouver was that the role and responsibility of hosting medical and therapy staff and providing care for athletes from around the world was taken very seriously. From the planning phases through delivery, we, as "hosts," listened and tried to provide what the visiting therapists needed, rather than what we thought they needed. The volunteer staff was trained to be responsive and customer service oriented, which is often forgotten in the busy world of sports medicine and therapy. By using our host team's expert knowledge in therapy care for international sports, listening to our guests and their needs, and integrating all professionals seamlessly together in the polyclinic, the environment that was created was described by many involved as "Medical Disneyland," and described by the International Olympic Committee (IOC) as one of the best polyclinics ever!

Planning for the games

As with any of these ventures, what starts as a "Sure, I'd be happy to do it" quickly develops into the feeling that "This will be a lot of work." To successfully care for more than 40,000 individuals in the Olympic family, one must start the planning phase early—ideally at least 3 years prior to the games themselves. In fact, many have referred to the provision of services to the athletes as 80% planning and 20% games involvement.

Sports Therapy Services, First Edition. Edited by James E. Zachazewski and David J. Magee.
© 2012 International Olympic Committee. Published 2012 by John Wiley & Sons, Ltd.

The initial step in the planning of how to host the games from a therapy perspective was to determine who would be the director of therapy services. It is essential that this individual has significant organizational skills, experience in professional meetings, excellent leadership qualities, considerable experience in attending and hosting international sporting events, and a very good working relationship with the chief medical officer (CMO). This interaction with the CMO is critical to the success of the program. The CMO must understand and support the important role that therapy plays in the recovery and regeneration of elite level athletes and their ability to compete.

Initially, the director of therapy services must have significant involvement in the planning process to help, guide, and develop a comprehensive needs assessment for therapy services including reviewing previous games data and being very involved with the organizing committee to ensure that the needs and requirements to provide world-class therapy care is considered. Often venue managers do not think about any medical topics until it is too late, and it is much easier to be involved early in the process to design space and to establish appropriate protocols and to ensure proper equipment is available where needed. It must be determined what venues require on-site therapy services, the location and size of the polyclinic therapy services in the athlete villages, as well as areas for *recovery and regeneration* (discussed in further detail later). Each location that is to have therapy provision must have a clearly defined role. For example, are the therapists or other medically related individuals providing immediate on-field care? Early definitions of qualifications required by volunteer staff will also help in the recruitment process so that there are clear "rules" on who will be eligible to volunteer. The director of therapy also must be visible in both the local community and the national professional communities early to develop excitement and clarity as to how people will be involved and how they can get involved. All of this planning involves many hours, and therefore, if one has the privilege of experiencing this role, one must also negotiate enough compensation to offset loss of income. Today, it is common practice that the leadership team be compensated, if not hired on a full-

time basis. The head of therapy services for a major games should be a full-time position, with one or two paid part-time assistants who operate as village polyclinic therapy managers. In the 2010 Games, the director of therapy services was a full-time position, and the polyclinic and venue supervisors of therapy received a small honorarium for their services.

Understanding the therapy needs

There is a saying "You don't know where you are going until you know where you have been!" The saying applies in this situation as well. Until recently, there has been a scarcity of information on the quantity and type of injuries managed at major games. While transfer of knowledge was preached and desired, once the games were over, things closed pretty quickly and most people wanted to be "done" and to get back to their normal lives. It is imperative that data is obtained throughout the games while things are happening to get a comprehensive idea of what services were delivered and whether they met the needs of the athlete and visiting teams.

The host medical committee for the Vancouver Olympic and Paralympic Games, as well as the IOC, kept excellent statistics for the 2010 Games using computerized tracking systems to monitor injuries both at the venues as well as in the polyclinics in the athlete villages. This was a daunting task that required the commitment of both the national organizing committees and their medical staff as well as the local host medical committee of the 2010 Games. Engebretsen *et al.* (2010) presented an excellent review of the data on athlete injuries from the 2010 Winter Olympic Games. Their data concludes that at least 11% of the athletes incurred an injury during the games, while 7% of the athletes experienced an illness. Junge *et al.* (2006) who were the first to conduct injury surveillance at the Beijing Olympic Games concluded that 10% of the athletes were injured at those games.

It is important to remember, however, that host medical services are responsible for the entire Olympic "family," which includes not only the athletes but also the coaches, officials, national sport organizations, media, sponsors, VIPs, and the workforce. While the therapy services provided must be athlete centered, it is important to realize the large potential for therapy needs when this larger group is considered. At the Vancouver 2010 Olympics, the therapy staff was responsible for the potential care of 7000 athletes, coaches, and officials, as well as 10,000 media and 25,000 volunteers and the workforce. There were 12 venues and training sites to cover, as well as three hotels for media and IOC officials, and two polyclinics in the athlete villages. According to the Summary of Medical Encounters for the 2010 Olympic Games, there were 8198 medical encounters for accredited individuals (e.g., Olympic family) and 840 spectator encounters. Twenty-nine percent (2621) of these encounters were related to the musculoskeletal system. These numbers were relatively consistent with the limited information received from previous winter games.

At the 2010 Olympic Games, therapy was provided at six venue sites as well as the two polyclinics in the athlete villages. As the name suggests, polyclinics are large spaces with dedicated areas for many subspecialties of care (e.g., therapy, medicine, dental, and ophthalmology). In the two village polyclinics, there were 1657 therapy sessions over the 26 days of the games. More than 50% of these visits were initial assessments and the average visits per day was 63.7 (Celebrini *et al.* 2010). The heaviest number of visits was from days 10 to 12 of the games. More specifics on the therapy will be provided later in the chapter.

One of the growing areas of interest in sporting communities is recovery and regeneration from training and competition. In recent years, therapy tubs, postevent massage, foam rollers, and restorative exercise have become more prevalent. In fact, this will be, in all likelihood, an area of increased interest and research over the next 10 years. The therapy group felt it was imperative to give the athletes and visiting medical/training staff this equipment to help them in their quest for ideal recovery. This area was located in close proximity to the therapy area in the polyclinics and included hot/cold therapy tubs, a stretching and cools down area, spin bikes, foam rollers, tubing, and other functional equipment such as medicine balls and proprioceptive equipment. At the 2010 Olympic Games, these

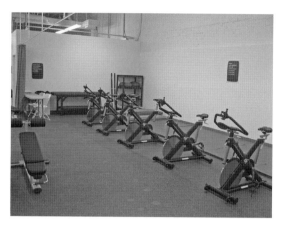

Figure 4.1 Recovery and regeneration area at 2010 Olympic Games

recovery and regeneration tools were actually located in the fitness facilities in the villages, which happened to be next to the polyclinics (Figure 4.1). Massage therapists were allocated as needed to this area and the areas could also be booked by a team to use privately by their own staff. One thousand and eighty-seven athletes used this area in the Vancouver athlete village.

Following a review of the needs and the plans that had to be delivered to provide the best therapy ever, the next step was to think about who was needed to deliver the care.

Getting the right people

The success of any team rests among the members of that team. There must be strong, respectful leadership, and egos must be "parked at the door." As mentioned previously, the team starts with an excellent leader called the director of therapy services. The next individuals to be brought into the process should be the supervisors of therapy services in the polyclinics in the Athlete Village. These individuals will play a major role in the organization and delivery of care to the majority of the Olympic family. They will act as the liaisons and "therapy ambassadors" with the other professions in the polyclinic. As well, they function as assistants to the director of therapy services in the organization of every aspect of therapy of the games (e.g., equipment,

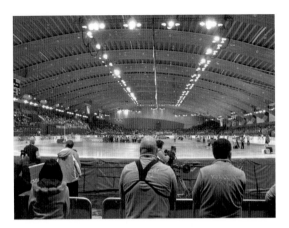

Figure 4.2 Speed skating venue at the 2010 Olympic Games

staffing, and medical records). It is imperative these individuals have a diverse background in sports therapy and have attended numerous events at the international level, both as a host and traveling therapist. Another necessary asset is that these individuals have experience managing multidisciplinary clinics in multiple locations. These organizational skills and multitasking abilities helped manage the most challenging situation of having two polyclinics. The supervisors are required to discuss and monitor ongoing change in a professional and calm manner. Everyday experience in planning, staff management, inventory management, and even marketing will help them lead their teams and the entire group effectively.

Each venue requires a supervisor of therapy services to oversee the delivery of care at that sport facility (Figure 4.2). These individuals should have specific international experience in the sports that are competing at the venue, both as a host therapist and a traveling therapist. Again experience as a team leader or clinic manager/owner would be an asset, and it is imperative that they develop a relationship with the sport. These individuals must be available in the year prior to the major games to be venue supervisor positions for test events. This establishes them as the "go to" person for the sport technical officials, as well as providing experience in developing protocols for the particular venue in immediate injury management and provision of care. It cannot be stressed enough how important

it is to have the majority of the entire team providing athlete care in place for these test events to "test" the team, provide planning, and to discuss, time and use of equipment, before the pressure and scrutiny of the major games occurs.

Along with recruiting of the major team members is the establishment of a support team for the director of therapy services. This includes an administrative assistant who is likely shared with a few of the other key medical personnel. In today's world, an information technology consultant is also essential. These individuals are the vital link in communication with the group as it begins to expand to the volunteer workforce.

The next step in the process is to determine what services will be provided at both the venues and the polyclinics. At the 2010 Olympic Games, it was decided that the therapy team would include physiotherapists, massage therapists, and athletic therapists. As well, it was decided to include chiropractors on the team. In the past, it was more common for chiropractors to provide care outside of the regular therapy team. However, it was decided for Vancouver that in order to provide a cohesive group for all individuals who needed care, chiropractors should be part of the team.

Each individual therapist was required to be eligible for licensure in British Columbia as well as have the necessary professional postgraduate certification such as diploma in sports physiotherapy or certification in sports massage. This requirement was to ensure competence from nationally recognized, examined certification as well as demonstrate the committee's support to continuing education and certification within the respective professions. International participants were required to have an equivalent certification from their country. Early in the planning process, a key person from each profession was identified to function as the liaison/supervisor of their individual profession (e.g., supervisor of massage therapy). This person assisted in working with the professional governing bodies, identifying potential talent within their profession, and communicating with their profession. These particular individuals were a real asset in helping to identify equipment needed and various specific requirements of their professions.

Through consultation with the visiting national sport organizations and their medical teams prior to the games, it was felt that acupuncture services should also be available, as well as bracing, hand therapy specialists, and orthotics. While none of these individuals were needed on a full-time basis, the need was identified and on call, or booked for limited hours on certain days in the polyclinics. The need for experts in specific fields of care was identified to be available on a consultation in areas such as electrotherapy, manual therapy, and whiplash-associated disorders. In Vancouver, it was fortunate that local individuals who are internationally recognized were available on a consultant basis. Needs were looked at from a traveling therapist point of view and questions were often raised in the meetings as to what services might be required by a traveling team from another country. While teams that have their own therapists will likely provide their own care, often they may need equipment maintenance, treatment advice on complicated problems, or someone to make an orthotic, build a hand splint, or have a knee brace fixed. The on-call consultants filled this need.

As the requirements for specific care were identified, the various professional groups were contacted to help get the message out about who qualified and what the volunteer opportunities were. This was done at national professional meetings by the director of therapy services, as well as through professional journals and newsletters. The therapy services administrative group worked closely with the professional colleges of each profession to ensure the appropriate licensure and malpractice insurance requirements were explained. This requirement was more complicated for international individuals, but as it was done early in the process, it led to much less stress for all involved. Calls were then put out for volunteers to apply to participate in the therapy coverage of the games asking them to indicate if they had a preference for a various area, but with the understanding that all preferences could not be met and clinicians would have to be flexible to enable the organizing group to fill particular needs and they would be placed where the needs were. Fortunately, there were very few situations that did not meet the desires of the team members. The volunteers were required to be

available for 2 weeks during the games as well as to attend one of the test events at the venue where they wanted to work. This ensured appropriate numbers of staff so that people did not burn out, and the test events started the team building and individual evaluation process early before the games began. Volunteers were required to provide their own transportation to the games, as well as arrange lodging; however, the local committee helped connect volunteers with local therapists or families prepared to house them for the duration of the games. The volunteers were also instructed that they would be required to purchase tickets to watch events at the games when they were not working. It was important to get this information out early to the team to provide them a chance to purchase tickets when they went on sale.

Once the applications to work as part of the host medical team were received, the applications were sorted to narrow the numbers to individuals who actually qualified to work at the games. The goal was to build teams for the venues and the polyclinics that had complimentary skill sets. Obviously, in the venues, immediate care skills were necessary. In the polyclinics, individuals with multiple skill training were an asset and various different skills were needed (e.g., chiropractors or massage therapists with active release therapy certification, physiotherapists with manual therapy skills or taping and bracing experience). In addition, a balance between males and females was considered as some countries still request a male or female therapist or massage therapist and as the host organization, it was important to provide services to everyone regardless of their beliefs. The global spirit of the Olympics was represented by ensuring our team members were from a variety of Canadian provinces as well as having some international members including therapists from the United States, Australia, and Brazil. As part of the legacy of the games, some of the more recently certified members of each profession were invited to be involved to give them experience at major games. It was the organizing committee's hope that this would encourage them to continue to be involved and foster the next generation of host therapists.

When selecting the candidates, each venue supervisor was consulted as well as the two polyclinic managers, and the teams were set. Then, at the test events, the needs of each area were reviewed as well as individuals attending the event were evaluated to see if they met the standards that had been set internally for people to be part of the "world-class" Vancouver team.

Having the right tools to do the job

As the recruiting process was being conducted, many hours were spent trying to work with the venue supervisors as well as the polyclinic managers to identify required equipment and supplies. Essentially, 10–12 therapy clinics were being created to be set up in a few days, run at maximum production for 10–30 days, and then torn down in a matter of a few days. Transfer of knowledge from previous games was a huge help in this area to determine supplies needed. Examples of this are the need for a competent large volume towel service as well as having an adequate constant supply of ice. At the 2010 Games, the medical services committee began working early with the games organizing committee to identify how these two items, that were problems at previous games, would be handled from a logistic point of view. With the appropriate planning, neither of these supply items was an issue in Vancouver.

One of the best early steps the Vancouver 2010 leadership team did was to ask their experienced therapy venue leaders to list equipment they thought would be needed. This process helped in thinking of all of the things possible, including various profession-specific tools. Once all the potential needs were listed, it became a challenge to determine "needs" versus "wants" within a budget. It is again important to do this process early so that there is plenty of time to seek sponsorship and donation of equipment and supplies. This list was separated into therapy equipment and therapy supplies (consumables) (Figure 4.3).

From an equipment standpoint, one must think about what the host therapists will use, as well as what the international community will be using. An example of this is shockwave therapy. While still in its early use clinically in Canada, this modality is used commonly in some European countries, and

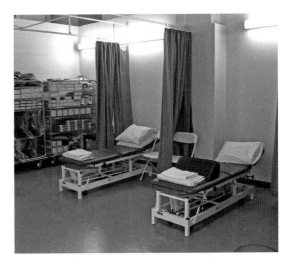

Figure 4.3 Equipment and supplies at the Vancouver Therapy Clinic at the 2010 Olympic Games

therefore it was felt that one should be available for the visiting therapists to use. As well, this was an excellent opportunity for the manufacturer to educate North American therapists on use of their equipment. A major games is an excellent opportunity for manufacturers to expose their equipment to a large number of elite therapists, coaches, athletes, and physicians. In return for this exposure, they should be willing to loan equipment for use at the games. While it may require some entrepreneurial creativity to work out an agreement of sponsorship, this can be achieved. Manufacturers may request other things such as marketing and any agreement must be cleared with the major games procurement department to ensure the rules are followed and not infringing on other sponsorship agreements. An individual with business savvy and experience in the sponsorship relationships is a huge asset to the team. For a complete list of the equipment in the polyclinic at the 2010 Games, see Table 4.1. All of the equipment listed in Table 4.1 was donated. The major donors had an opportunity to educate the therapists on the use of their equipment during the games. This had the additional benefit of the team members learning current research and application involving the different pieces of equipment.

The second list that needed to be created was a list of "consumable" therapy supplies required.

Table 4.1 Therapy equipment

Quantity	Equipment	Quantity	Equipment
1	Electrotherapy Combo and Cart: TENS, IFC, HVPC, ultrasound, EMG, laser, Russian, diadynamic	1	7.5″ Plyometric/Medicine Ball 4 kg (8.8 lbs) blue
1	Ultrasound unit	1	7.5″ Plyometric/Medicine Ball 6 kg (13.2 lbs) green
2	TENS unit	5	Various sized exercise balls
1	High volt unit	2	Dumbbells—2 lbs
3	Muscle stimulation unit	2	Dumbbells—3 lbs
1	EMG	2	Dumbbells—5 lbs
1	Biofeedback—EMG	2	Dumbbells—8 lbs
2	Stabilizer pressure biofeedback cuffs	2	Dumbbells—10 lbs
1	Laser	1	Dumbbells—15 lbs
1	High volt/multistimulation combo unit	1	Dumbbells—20 lbs
1	IMS electrostimulator	9	Theraband/Theratubing (rolls)
1	Portable microcurrent device	5	Gymsticks
1	Hydrocollator heating unit (12 pack), including packs/covers	1	Reebok Coreboards
1	Game ready cryocuff system	1	Trampoline
1	Neurocryostim unit	1	Power Skater
1	Shortwave diathermy	3	Various wobble boards
2	Hi-Boy whirlpool 105 Gallon	2	Sissel discs
1	Cryo IR	1	Cuff weights (set 1–5 kg)
1	Shockwave ESWT and RSWT Mechanical Traction unit	1	Medicine ball rebounders
			Other
1	Treadmills	8	HI-Lo treatment tables, 1 chiropractic table
2	Upright Monark 928e	1	Therabath PRO Paraffin Bath w/6 1 lb bars
1	Vision Fitness 2750HRT "Step Through" recumbent bike	1	Jamar Hand Evaluation Set (3 pcs), each
		1	Flowin Pro Plate vibration plate
1	Arm ergometer	1	Wheel chair
1	Cable system	8	Exam stools, bolsters, therapy belts
1	Shuttle		*For Recovery Regeneration area*
2	Exercise mats	6	Ethoform Rounds/Styrofoam rolls
2	BOSU balance board	6	Stretch Cords/Rubber Rope 9 ft
1	Pro Fitter 3D Cross Trainer	5	Stretch Mats
1	7.5″ Plyometric/Medicine Ball 2 kg (4.4 lbs) red	6	Upright bikes
		2	Arm ergometers
		2	Softubs

Reproduced from Celebrini *et al.* (2010) with permission from Rick Celebrini.

These supplies were those products that would be consumed during the games and used in the delivery of care in the therapy clinics. Some of these supplies were, however, sometimes given out to a visiting therapist if needed. Table 4.2 provides a list of supplies for the village polyclinic. This list does not include the hand therapy-specific splinting supplies or orthotic supplies and braces as these items were achieved through a specific sponsorship relationship, and will be discussed further in the next section. The therapy supply items were largely supplied through donations, as manufacturers were keen to get their products in the hands of elite level therapists, and have elite level athletes try their product. If not donated completely, often a relationship was reached in which the supplier gave a discount in return for advertising/recognition as a donor.

Finally, it is important to have comprehensive lists of both the equipment and the supplies prior to the games. This will enable shipments to be monitored and inventory to be controlled and helps inventory checking when packing up at the end of the games.

Table 4.2 Therapy supplies

Actiflex Elastic Bandage 2″	Leukotape P, $1\frac{1}{2}″ \times 15$ yd
Actiflex Elastic Bandage 3″	Lister Bandage Scissors 7.25″
Actiflex Elastic Bandage 4″	Maunder Oral Screw
Actiflex Elastic Bandage 6″	Memory Foam Blue (Adhesive) 3/8″ × 16″ × 24″/Sheet
Airgo Lightweight Wheelchair (18 × 16)	Metatarsal Arch Pad-(Medium-3)
Aluminum Foam Finger Splints—0.5″ × 18″	Moleskin 3″ × 25 yd
Aluminum Foam Finger Splints 1″ × 18″	Moleskin, Latex Free
Ambufix Splint	Mueller Heel and Lace Pads
Ankle Brace w/Stays	Mueller Knee Strap—Black
Antimicrobial Hand Wipes	Mueller Massage Lotion—1 Gal
Bacitracin Ointment Foil Packs 0.9g	Non Adherent Gauze Pads 3″ × 4″
Back Support	NS, 15 cc, Pour
Bandage, Elast, 3″ (Tensor)	Orthogel Variety Pack
Bandage, Elast, 4″ (Tensor)	Ossur ROM—Universal
Beirsdorf Lightplast Pro Elastic Tape 2″ × 7.5 yd	Paper Cups
Beirsdorf Lightplast Pro Elastic Tape 3″ × 7.5 yd	Paramed Utility Scissors 8″
Bunga Pads	Patella Knee Support
Bunga Pads	Petroleum Jelly
Chattanooga Utility Cart, Plastic, Black—3 Shlv	Positex Mobilization Strap (8 ft)
Clinton Exam Stool—Model 2102	Powerflex AFD 4″ × 2.5 yd, Sterile
Com-Pressor SI Belt	Rapid Relief Instant Cold Pack 5″ × 9″
Cramer High Density Foam Kit	Safety Pin
Cramer Ice Bags $9\frac{1}{2}″ \times 18″$	Sam Splint—Charcoal
Cramer Shark Tape Cutter	Saunders Shoulder Brace
Cramer Skin Lube 1 lb	Spenco 2nd Skin—1″ Squares
Cramer Tape Remover 1 pt.	Splinter Forceps—$4\frac{1}{2}″$
Cramergesic 1 lb	StimTrode 2″ ×2″ Pre-Gelled Cloth Backed
Crutches—Aluminum Adult Xtra Tall	StimTrode 2″ ×3.5″ Pre-Gelled Cloth Backed
Dexidin—4% Chlorhexidine (450 mL)	Super Pro 11 Scissors (Metal)
Disposable Arm Sling	Table Paper, smooth, 18″ × 225″
Double Length Elastic Bandage 6″	Tape Underwrap
Elbow Support	Taylor Percussion Hammer
Felt Variety Pack—Assorted	Tensoplast Non-Rippable Elastic Tape 2″ × $5\frac{1}{2}$ yd
Fingernail Clippers—Pocket Size	Tensoplast Non-Rippable Elastic Tape 3″ × $5\frac{1}{2}$ yd
Flexall Extra Strength—7 lb	Thigh Sleeve-Neoprene
Flex-I-Wrap w/Handle 4″	Thumb Guard
Foam Corn Pads C6	Toenail Clippers Pocket Size (L)
Foam Foot Donuts, Grey	Tuli's Pro Heel Cup (Large)
Forearm Crutch	Tuli's Pro Heel Cups (Regular)
Functional Wrist Support	Vaseline Skin Lotion (525 mL)
Gauze Bandage Rolls Nonsterile 3″ × 4.1 yd	Visine Eye Drops (15 mL)
Gauze Bandage Rolls Sterile 2″ × 4.1 yd	White Swan Mini-Wipes
Gauze Bandage Rolls Sterile 4″ × 4.1 yd	Wrist Splint
Goniometer—Plastic 12″	Oral Airway, 100 mm (Red)
Goniometer—Plastic 6″	Oral Airway, 80 mm (Green)
Hinged Knee Brace	Oral Airway, 90 mm (Yellow)
J&J Coach Athletic Tape $1\frac{1}{2}″$	Oxygen—Bag-Valve Mask—Adult
J&J Orthoplast II 18 × 24″ Plain (1 sheet)	Abdominal Pad, 5″ × 9″
J&J Zonas Athletic Tape 1″	Abdominal Pad, 5″ × 9″
KineMedics—T2	Abdominal Pad, 5″ × 9″
Knee Immobilizer, Universal, 24″	Bandage, Elast, 3″ (Tensor)
Knee Sleeve—Open Patella	Bandage, Elast, 3″ (Tensor)
Leukostrip 6.4 mm × 102 mm 5/pkg	Bandage, Elast, 3″ (Tensor)

Table 4.2 (*Continued*)

Band-Aids Dressing	SAM Splint, 4 × 18″
Band-Aids Dressing	Sponge, Gauze, 2 × 2 (Sterile)
Band-Aids Dressing	Sponge, Gauze, 2 × 2 (Sterile)
Blue Bin	Sponge, Gauze, 2 × 2 (Sterile)
Blue Bin	Sponge, Gauze, 4 × 4 (Bulk)
Blue Bin	Sponge, Gauze, 4 × 4 (Bulk)
Conform Bandage, 3″	Sponge, Gauze, 4 × 4 (Bulk)
Conform Bandage, 3″	Tape, Transpore, 1″ (IV Clear)
Conform Bandage, 3″	Tape, Transpore, 1″ (IV Clear)
NS, 500 cc, Pour	Tape, Transpore, 1″ (IV Clear)
NS, 500 cc, Pour	Telfa Dressing, 3″ × 4″
NS, 500 cc, Pour	Telfa Dressing, 3″ × 4″
SAM Splint, 4 × 18″	Telfa Dressing, 3″ × 4″
SAM Splint, 4 × 18″	

Reproduced from Celebrini *et al.* (2010) with permission from Rick Celebrini.

Communication is key

Major sports games are massive undertakings, and each component of the organization must understand what sports therapists do and what they need to be successful. The therapy area is one of the busiest in the polyclinics, as well as in the village. Facility design people must know how much space is needed, as well as why such things as open areas for exercise, private rooms are needed. The supply chain must understand why ice and clean towels are needed. The various members of the polyclinic team including physicians, diagnostic imaging, nursing, and administration need to understand what therapists do and what their role is. One of the most successful components of the Vancouver experience was two major meetings held prior to the games that brought all facets of the polyclinics together to explain what they do, how they were going to deliver their service at the games, and challenges they would face. These meetings helped everyone understand the various professions and got the group working together. Therapy-specific meetings were also held to put all the leadership members of our team together to discuss each therapy profession's needs and how excellence in each area of therapy was going to be achieved.

With e-mail, communication to the therapy team was much easier. Upon selection, each team member was sent forms electronically to complete on immunization requirements, licensing instructions, information about the games, and even biographies of other team members. Therapy goals were clearly defined and the message stressed that what was being done was a team effort providing care and that "egos and professional political issues were to be left at home." Every individual had something to contribute and all therapists had an opportunity to experience a once-in-a-lifetime event. Scheduling was done quite easily using Excel® so that each team member had a finalized schedule well in advance of the games so they could book plane flights and accommodation. Even last minute schedule changes could be handled by doing a mass e-mail to the group asking for help. This scheduling information was then included in the games staff database so the organizing committee knew exactly how many staff needed to be fed on certain days, and who was to be accredited for various time frames and venues. While the teams were kept as consistent as possible in one location, some therapists did work in both the clinic and venues. As the games drew closer, information was distributed by e-mail about such things as therapist accreditation and uniforms. The use of e-mail in this way was very successful.

Another important aspect of communication was patient charting and recording of interventions for analysis and information for future games. The 2010 Olympic Games used a limited computer charting system to register patients and link their file to their accreditation number. This file was then used to track their progress through the particular medical encounter. Notes could be added by the primary physician, nursing staff, diagnostic imaging, laboratory analysis, pharmacy, and therapy and could be updated on a daily basis if necessary. If the individual was treated at a venue, the information could be reviewed and added to in the polyclinic data. Even diagnostic imaging and ultrasound results at the venues could be transmitted electronically to be read by the experts in the polyclinic imaging departments. This software was the primary source for the medical encounter data presented in the literature from the games.

Unfortunately, the medical encounter software was designed by physicians for medicine and had limited information on types of therapy provided or specific charting requirements for therapists. Thus, it was decided to have a paper chart for each patient with therapy-specific charting, as well as a manual/computer system to track therapy statistics. While not ideal, this provided effective communication between therapists who were seeing the same patient on different days, and provided a very clear picture after the games of what services were used. Future hosts should consider the ability to have a fully integrated, multidisciplinary electronic medical records capability.

Finally, a computer system was used for scheduling patient visits, as well as scheduling the recovery/regeneration area. This program was set up to allow a certain number of visits per therapist, as well as how many therapists were available per day. It was linked to the front-office administration, so anyone who called the polyclinic could book an appointment with therapy without bothering the therapists. The therapists were trained to book follow-up appointments so they could schedule the appropriate amount of time without bothering the front desk again as it was quite a distance from the therapy area. This system was very effective and efficient.

It was also important to communicate with the national sport organizations to initially ask them what they required and then communicate how services would be delivered. Meeting with visiting medical teams at test events was vital. This included teams that would have their own staff at the games, as well as those that required heavier use of the host services for care. Following these initial "listening"

meetings and e-mails, regular communication was established with the CMO/chief therapists from all of the visiting countries to inform them of the services that would be provided as well as ongoing issues (e.g., H1N1 control, licensing of visiting professionals). There was also a fairly comprehensive manual published for each visiting team, prior to the games, on all the medical services provided and how they could be accessed. Communicating with all the stakeholders whether they are part of the internal games organization or visiting guests was fundamental to the Vancouver success of hosting the world.

Let the games begin

The finishing touches

Based on the Vancouver perspective and experience, after 3 years of planning everyone on the team was quite excited to be in the "home stretch." Years of talking were now a reality, and the games were days away. However, nothing in one's life will prepare anyone for the week leading up to the games. The week before the games, 40,000 people will descend on a community, each having their own role in the event. Finishing touches are still being done on the facilities, equipment is still arriving, therapy team members have hundreds of questions, and one must continue to work with all the facets of the organizing committee. The ability to work with a few hours of sleep, manage unexpected surprises, and having a good sense of humor is required.

With today's security challenges, the setup process at the venues and the clinics largely revolved around the needs of the police and safety officials. After final inspection of the empty facilities, there will be a rush to get equipment and supplies into the village before the "bomb sweep" and "lock down" of the village. This "move in" phase requires 3–4 days. It is essential to have accurate lists of what was to be delivered to each therapy location and have someone at the location to confirm it arrived. At this point, daily communication with each venue supervisor and the polyclinic managers is critical. Once the village is "locked down," all

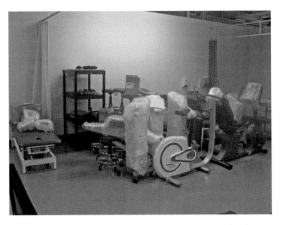

Figure 4.4 Therapy equipment to be unpacked

the supplies must go through an intensive screening process to get into the villages or competition therapy areas (Figure 4.4).

An example of adapting to a changing environment happened on the day unpacking of shipments was to start in the Vancouver Village Polyclinic. One of the bomb-sniffing dogs identified one of the paper shredders as being positive. This created an 8-hour delay, and the day of unpacking turned into an evening/night of frenzied activity to stay on schedule for the polyclinic opening. Fortunately, it was a false alarm, but the medical organizing committee must be prepared to handle such events and continue on.

As items are unpacked, they should be identified and recorded. To facilitate interdisciplinary/ professional collaboration in Vancouver, it was decided that rather than having separate areas for each profession, all professions would share all of the area/treatment space. This worked successfully and was one of the best ideas presented by one of our staff, as it delivered a true team environment.

It is important to have the manufacturers help set up their equipment especially if it is complicated and to have the individuals unpacking any equipment to be familiar with its basic construction to be able to assemble it if needed. Having a small tool kit in the clinics would be helpful to assemble and repair the equipment.

Once the equipment is set up and arranged in its location, biomedical technicians should ensure

that the equipment was calibrated and operating safely. The technicians are usually outside individuals who required temporary accreditation. Operation of hot and cold tubs in the recovery area should be inspected by local health officials for water quality and to review the sanitization/chemical process before allowing anyone to use the tubs/pools. The tubs/pools should be inspected regularly during the games. Logbooks are required to record when the chemicals have been checked and adjusted.

Finally, the supplies are unpacked and put in their appropriate location. It is suggested that only a small amount of supplies actually be out in the open while the remainder are in a storeroom out of sight. This will provide inventory control against overuse and losses from theft. This also applies to all small electrotherapeutic devices such as TENS machines.

When designing the clinical space, one must remember to have a place for staff to put their personal belongings as well as an area for them to chart are required. The supervisor of the venue or clinic will need an area to do his/her assigned paperwork, or meet with individuals if required to discuss something confidentially. Finally, a signboard or white board in a prominent location was excellent for communicating the day's events or any other information for the entire therapy team. Once all the computers are networked and running properly, the clinic is organized, and the supplies recorded and stored, one is ready for the team to arrive and open the clinic to a gradual increase in traffic.

"Getting the team to gel"

The concept of "team building" is critical to the success of operations. One of the most consistent pieces of feedback received from the therapy staff after the Vancouver Games was "how much fun it was to work with a great team." This was gratifying to hear as considerable time and energy had been put into planning to bring the team of high-profile individuals together as a group. This plan was initiated on the first day the therapy team arrived, which was 1 day before the athletes and Olympic family began to arrive.

Orientation and education of staff are necessary and should be mandatory. Using the Vancouver 2010 Games as an example, Day 1 began with a large meeting of all of the volunteers from all of the departments in the polyclinics. A similar meeting occurred at each venue. This large meeting was chaired by the manager of the polyclinic as well as the supervisors. Since customer service was not often linked with health care, the concept of customer service was emphasized. Topics included acknowledging people in the immediate vicinity, defining what a host was, the "power of a smile," and other customer service approaches. Each supervisor then provided a brief overview of their service and emergency procedures were reviewed. Following the large meeting, each professional group was given a private tour of the polyclinic and had a meeting in their area to review therapy-specific items such as charting, a review of the clinical software, confidentiality, and other last minute details. An education session was then held by one of the polyclinic experts on current research in electrotherapy as well as giving our manufacturers an opportunity to explain their equipment (Figure 4.5). Finally, on-call services (i.e., orthotics, hand specialists, and brace company) provided an overview of the service and equipment they could provide. Refreshments were served and this day became an excellent day of training, sharing, and team bonding. This training day was repeated as

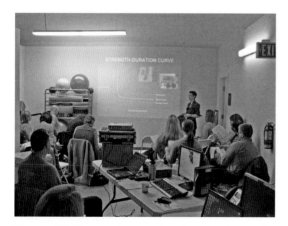

Figure 4.5 Therapy team education session at the 2010 Olympic Games

new staff came on board after the first group was finished their 2 weeks.

At the start of each shift, the supervisor should have a quick meeting with the new shift to discuss any changes in the procedure from the day before. While policies and procedures may be established before the start of the games, daily shift meetings such as this are critical as the operational rules are often being "written" as the games progressed day to day, resulting in minor changes in polyclinic procedures throughout the games. The supervisor also attended daily early morning polyclinic meetings to ensure the polyclinic as a whole was operating smoothly. A "team building" dinner was scheduled after the first week of working to encourage social interaction away from the clinic. Other projects to encourage communication such as a daily trivia question with a small prize and occasionally asking one of the team members to show the others one of their clinical tidbits and "pearls of wisdom." Informal case reviews were held if there was an interesting situation that arose and all of our team members embraced the concept that this was a great learning opportunity for all. The local organizing committee also provided occasional free event tickets to be given to staff who excelled at the "team" concept. Finally, a small space in the village, better known as the "Tiki lounge," served as a social post shift gathering area where medical friends, new and old, could relax after a shift.

To facilitate the therapy team working well with the others in the clinic (e.g., doctors, nurses, and diagnostic imaging technicians), clinicians were to be the first person to communicate. In Vancouver, the therapy team made a distinct effort to introduce themselves to the general practitioners and sport medicine physicians who were doing the triage in the clinic, because it was felt to be essential to the success that they understand what therapists did. The supervisor took the time to meet each physician individually on their first shift and explain the services that could be provided. Each team member took the time to explain what they were doing if another professional was being toured through the clinical area. If the team had time, they were encouraged to go and meet someone from another profession, and all of the professions embraced this concept to share and learn. It got to the point that individuals did not want to end their shift because they were afraid to miss something. Even our on-call people would come into the clinic just to see what was being discussed or taught. This resulted in a group that worked hard when they needed to and had fun learning when there was a spare moment.

Welcoming the world to our facility

Once the space was organized and everything was in place, the team was ready to welcome the world. Each visiting medical team was invited to come for a tour of the polyclinic as they arrived, once they had settled into their temporary home. In Vancouver, almost all of the teams took the time to come and find out what services were available. This was an excellent opportunity for the supervisor of therapy services to meet the visiting therapists, explain the services available, as well as to let the visiting therapists know that if they needed anything they could call on the clinic and help would be available. Future games schedules should be set up so that the supervisor has time to do this important role, as it was felt to be critical to our success of hosting. The traveling therapy teams were visited in their temporary clinics in the village to ensure that all of their equipment worked for them and that they knew where to get ice/towels and other things they needed. This first contact was crucial to establish the partnership between visiting therapists and the hosts to provide the best care possible for their athletes. If the visiting country did not have therapists with them, some time was spent with the medical officer to explain how therapy/medical services could be accessed and review the referral process. As with any major games, there were times when the translation services provided by the organizing committee were used to make our communication effective.

Once the majority of teams arrived, there was a reception planned by the host medical/therapy group to welcome all the visiting medical teams to Canada. This was again an opportunity to present the team's desire to help, the procedures for getting things done, and to help develop friendly networking among all the traveling and host therapists and other medical personnel. As the games progressed,

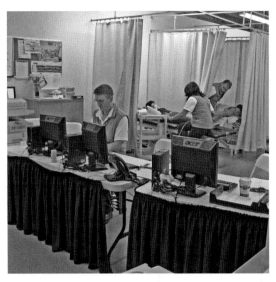

Figure 4.6 Functioning therapy clinic at the 2010 Olympic Games

the supervisor of therapy services often checked with the teams head therapist to ensure things were going well and make sure they were pleased with the services provided. Throughout the games, the IOC also hosted three, well attended, education sessions for all medical staff in the villages. These sessions featured international experts on topics such as the diagnosis and treatment of neck injuries and concussions.

The therapy clinic was open from 7:00 AM until 11:00 PM (Figure 4.6). This translated into two 8-hour shifts of staff. Each shift had two to three physiotherapists, three massage therapists, and one chiropractor. One massage therapist was designated per shift to be responsible for the recovery/regeneration area and, if not needed there, provided overflow coverage in the clinic area. This level of staffing was sufficient for the patient load, as well as having therapists able to take breaks. Each shift had one individual, chosen by the supervisor, to be the "torchbearer" of the shift. They would help delegate the caseload if needed, and be an assistant supervisor if needed. This responsibility was rotated throughout the team members during the games. The bracing companies who had their product available for use had an individual on call for fitting advice. As well, the on-call orthotics and hand specialists were available within 2 hours of the call

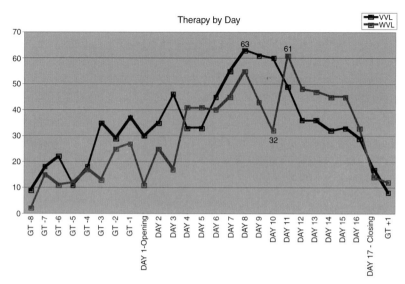

Figure 4.7 Daily use of therapy services at the 2010 Olympic Games. VVL, Vancouver Village Clinic; WVL, Whistler Village Clinic (Reproduced from Celebrini *et al.* (2010) with permission from Rick Celebrini.)

during clinic hours. An acupuncturist was available each evening, as well as on call during the day.

The actual number and types of therapy visits in each of the polyclinics at the 2010 Olympic Games was fairly similar. A total of 1657 physiotherapy sessions were provided over the course of a 26-day period for an average of 63.7 visits per day between the two polyclinics (does not include venues). Data was collected 8 days before games time (GT −8) to 1 day after the games closed (GT +1). Of the 1657 visits, 880 (53.1%) were at the Vancouver village (VVL) and 777 (46.9%) at the Whistler village (WVL) (Figure 4.7).

Fifty-two percent of the visits were athletes while the remainder were Olympic family members. Seven hundred and sixty of these visits were new assessments and the spine was the most common area of treatment, followed by knees and shoulders. Thirty-seven percent of the visits were provided by physiotherapists while 43% of the visits were massage. Chiropractors treated 16% of the visits and acupuncture and on-call specialties accounted for 2% each. Given the data, for future games, chiropractors, due to the limited demand for their specific services, could be an on-call profession with scheduled evening appointments.

Table 4.3 shows a breakdown of therapy service by modality and treatment techniques used. The busiest times of the day in the clinics were from 7:00 to 10:00 AM and from 6:00 to 10:00 PM.

The use of the clinic by athletes presented some interesting data as shown in Figure 4.8. While the two countries that used the services the most, Denmark and Ukraine, had minimal support services of their own, Canada was the third largest user of host services in the Vancouver village. This is probably due to the significant national team experience of many of the clinic therapists and their relationship with athletes attending the games. As well, there was a seamless relationship with the Canadian team core medical staff and our host therapy staff, with the polyclinic providing some care while the dedicated therapist was at the competition venue.

One of the interesting situations that occurred with athletes from other countries coming to see the clinic therapists was their wanting the fact that they had been to the clinic to be confidential. Fortunately, this did not present in a "return to play" situation and was more an aspect of the athlete getting a second opinion of the type of care he/she was receiving.

Table 4.3 Breakdown of therapy services

	VVL	WVL	Total		VVL	WVL	Total
Electrical stimulation devices				*Other*			
NMES	4	64	68	Deep Muscle Stim	4	3	7
TENS	3	4	7	Acupuncture (by physios)	18	16	34
Iontophoresis	0	0	0	IMS (by physios)	1	45	46
IFC	22	28	50	Mechanical traction	6	4	10
RUS	1	2	3	*Total*	*29*	*68*	*97*
HVG	0	2	2	*Assistive devices*			
Total	*30*	*100*	*130*	Taping	63	18	81
Therapeutic radiation device				Bracing (by physiotherapists)	22	112	134
Laser	28	25	53	Splinting	3	4	7
Total	*28*	*25*	*53*	Orthotics	1	1	2
Electromagnetic therapy device				Crutches	5	20	25
Shortwave	10	2	12	*Total*	*94*	*155*	*249*
Total	*10*	*2*	*12*	*Exercise*			
Sound energy devices				Proprioceptive	54	50	104
Ultrasound	92	85	177	Strength	74	65	139
Shockwave ES	1	15	16	Range of motion	132	110	242
Total	*93*	*100*	*193*	Gait	12	8	20
Superficial heating agents				Biofeedback	5	0	5
Hot Pack	55	65	120	Functional movement	52	56	108
Wax	5	2	7	Other (posture, education, etc.)	33	29	62
Total	*60*	*67*	*127*	*Total*	*362*	*318*	*680*
Cryotherapy agents				*Manual therapy*			
Cold Pool	5	0	5	Joint mobilization	292	264	556
Ice	36	41	77	Joint manipulation	156	152	308
Cryocuff	24	20	44	Stretch	201	185	386
Total	*65*	*61*	*126*	Manual traction	97	83	180
				ART	53	40	93
				Myofascial Rx	57	60	117
				Other (Mulligan, graston, etc.)	33	28	61
				Total	*889*	*812*	*1701*

Reproduced from Celebrini *et al.* (2010) with permission from Rick Celebrini.
ART, active release therapy; VVL, Vancouver Village Clinic; WVL, Whistler Village Clinic.

The amount of use of the therapy service and in fact the whole polyclinic during the games by athletes and Olympic family was a surprise. Likely due to the economy at the time, some of the larger teams did not have many therapists with them and this resulted in overflow to the polyclinic therapists. As word spread at the outstanding level of care being provided, it became a must see even for international dignitaries and future games hosts. The therapy clinic was very busy and was a hub of treatment and educational activity, often with impromptu in services erupting as one of the staff explained a technique they were using.

The 3 weeks of the games flew by and was culminated with Canada winning the gold medal in hockey and spectacular closing ceremonies. Many international friends were made and there was a very strong feeling of helping each and every athlete (or Olympic family member) who accessed the service with the best outcome-based level of care possible in the world.

Following the games

When the games concluded, another rush of activity and work ensued. The first step started on

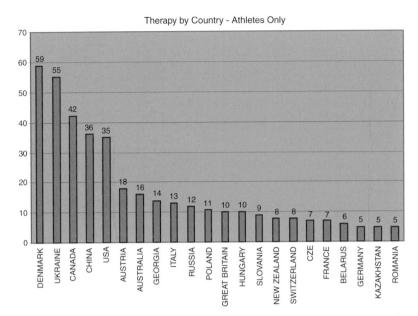

Figure 4.8 Use of therapy services by athlete/country in Vancouver Village Polyclinic (Reproduced from Celebrini *et al.* (2010) with permission from Rick Celebrini.)

the evening of the closing ceremonies. Athletes were keen to have a personal memento of their experience, so all moveable items needed to be locked up. Each volunteer in our group received a personal gift and thank-you for participating in the games. Once the athletes had left, the teardown began. This is when the lists that were made from the "move in" process become essential. The move out requires inventory taking, packing up all the supplies and equipment, and making sure they are properly labeled and packaged together to return to the appropriate supplier or sponsor. Data from the statistics collected is compiled and then reports are completed to pass on the knowledge to the next games.

Each volunteer from the team was contacted following the games to determine three things that made the event special for them. The consensus of this survey was the mutual respect of all professions to learn and listen to each other and that the provision of patient-centered care was essential to the host clinic's success. The educational sessions helped bring the learning environment to the fore-

front, and the strong, experienced, open leadership fostered a positive feeling throughout the team. It was truly one of the best experiences in our professional careers.

References

Celebrini, R., Stewart, R., Froese, A. *et al.* (2010) Summary of medical encounter data during the Vancouver 2010 Olympic and Paralympic Winter Games, August 2010.

Engebretsen, L., Steffen, K., Alonso, J. *et al.* (2010) Sports injuries and illnesses during the Winter Olympic Games 2010. *British Journal of Sports Medicine*, 44, 772–780.

Junge, A., Langevoort, G. & Pipe, A. (2006) Injuries in team sport tournaments during the 2004 Olympic Games. *American Journal of Sports Medicine*, 34, 565–576.

Webster's Dictionary on-line, http://www.merriam-webster.com/dictionary/host, February 2011.

Chapter 5
Pre-Olympic team travel: logistical and treatment considerations

Masaki Katayose[1] and David J. Magee[2]

[1]Sapporo Medical University, Sapporo, Hokkaido, Japan
[2]University of Alberta, Edmonton, AB, Canada

Introduction

Prior to the Olympic Games, athletes and coaches have many challenging issues that must be dealt with to ensure the athletes have had the best preparation and are at the peak of their performance when competing at the Olympic Games. The strategies for dealing with these issues may be diverse; however, sports therapists must help prepare each team and each athlete to accomplish their ultimate goal—success at the Olympics. For this chapter, the primary author is the chief therapist of the Japanese delegation to the two Olympic Games in Salt Lake City and Turin and also a medical support subcommission member of the Japanese Olympic Committee (JOC). The secondary author has attended three Olympics, numerous world aquatic championships, and several other major games, acting as a therapist for the host country and as a member of the country's delegation at other games. They will explain the sports therapy considerations for team travel prior to an Olympic Games.

Pre-event training camp

Prior to an Olympic Games, most athletes and coaches are well prepared physiologically and psychologically. Their training programs have been paced to achieve the highest level of performance at the Olympics. Their training program will have involved physiological issues such as periodization and peaking at the appropriate time. To help the athlete reach his or her maximum potential and to develop team spirit and rapport between team members, and to train under environmental conditions (i.e., weather, altitude) similar to where the Olympic Games will be held, most teams will hold a training camp for their athletes for 1–2 months before the games to help the athletes become acclimatized to their surroundings. Thus, the support team, including the sports therapist(s), must gather information on available facilities for both training and lodging, and environmental information when determining where any training camps will be held. This is especially true for things that could

Sports Therapy Services, First Edition. Edited by James E. Zachazewski and David J. Magee.
© 2012 International Olympic Committee. Published 2012 by John Wiley & Sons, Ltd.

affect performance at the Olympic Games such as altitude, humidity, temperature, and other factors such as lodging, eating, security, and sanitary conditions that could affect the well-being and safety of the athletes.

Ideally, someone (or several people) will arrange for and complete a reconnaissance visit to the training camp location several months beforehand to ensure the needs of the team are met. This reconnaissance team will determine such things as suitable accommodation and meals, where training and competition facilities are, how the facilities may be accessed, level of security available and needed, and to ensure there is appropriate equipment for team members to use for practice and training. It is very important for athletes to be given sufficient time to acclimatize and to adapt their physical condition to the geographical and environmental conditions at the training and Olympic sites to ensure they can train and compete with maximum effectiveness. Acclimatization commonly takes from 10 days to 2 weeks.

Most Olympic athletes will also participate in various regular international games sponsored by their respective international federations such as FIS and FIFA, even though these competitions may occur in the same year as the Olympics. In some cases, the athletes have to participate in these games/events to get the world cup points, or to obtain a suitable level of performance to be able to achieve the minimum standard to be able to take part and compete at the Olympics.

Some athletes and teams will come to the Olympics from different locations and countries around the world, so it is important for the sport therapist to understand the effects of travel on the athletes' physical condition and performance and to recommend appropriate measures to ensure these effects on performance are kept to a minimum. Issues such as jet lag, dehydration, time zone changes, all of which can upset the athletes' circadian rhythms, must be taken into account.

Based on this background, a pre-event training camp may be arranged for individual teams (most common) or for a whole Olympic delegation. Some of these camps will be arranged in a local domestic area that has similar weather and altitude to where the games will be held and some will be held at international sites, depending on the strategy and desires of the coaches, athletes, teams, and officials. Domestic local areas are usually easier to set up because many of the logistical and organizational issues are much easier to work out. Training sites held at international sites commonly require more planning but have the advantage of allowing the athletes, in addition to physiological acclimatization, to acclimatize to the cultures and customs that are similar to where the games will be held provided the training camps are arranged close to the Olympic site.

Sports therapists need to understand the purpose of pre-event training camp as it relates to each team and each athlete. The primary role of the sports therapist is to advise the coaches and athletes on issues such as injury, illness, and other health-related issues that may affect the performance of the athletes and to treat any problems. As such, the sports therapist needs to have the medical history of the athletes and other team members before going to the training camp. In Japan, the JOC organizes medical and conditioning checkups for all of the athletes who may go to the Olympics, usually, twice a year. For example, in Japan, these are usually carried out in the Institute of Sports Science (JISS), which is the center to enhance the performance of Japanese top athletes with sports science, sports medicine, and sports intelligence (Figure 5.1). These checkups enable the team to determine the health status of the athlete and if any diseases are present and whether they are

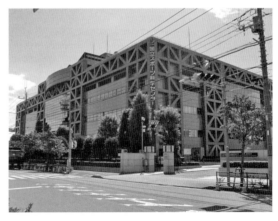

Figure 5.1 Japan Institute of Sports Sciences

amenable to treatment, preexisting conditions can be uncovered, baseline values can be established, a musculoskeletal profile and screening process can be developed, good health practices can be fostered, the athletes can be counseled if necessary (e.g., about doping, nutrition), and such screening can prevent a misinterpretation of findings later on. If such a medical history is not available, the sports therapist will have to contact a number of individuals (with the athlete's and team members' permission) to get this information. He or she will have to ensure the members of the team (both athletes and support personnel) have sufficient amounts of any medications they will need and to ensure the medications are checked to be sure they do not contravene any doping regulations.

In addition, the sports therapist must ensure the safety of the athletes by inspecting the practice and training sites to ensure there are no issues that may affect the health and safety of the athlete or any other team member (e.g., holes in the practice field, stationary objects close to the training surface that the athletes could run into). He or she should look for emergency exits at the training sites, location and distance of the nearest hospital, the services provided or available at this hospital, and how the services accessed would need to be paid for. Sanitation at the training and lodging sites and methods of communication available between team members at all locations are also important issues that must be determined.

With an understanding of the teams needs, the sports therapist can arrange to have the appropriate medical equipment and supplies available for the camp. In most cases, provided appropriate funding is available, teams try to be "self-contained" so that they will travel with all the equipment they need. Most sports therapists also have much of their own equipment and supplies. This enables the sport therapist to have equipment and supplies he or she is familiar with to use when treating the athletes and other team members. It also ensures that the sports therapist has on hand the supplies and equipment he or she will need rather than have to look for a potential substitute that does not meet the needs of the sports therapist. If the decision is to have a training camp for the whole Olympic team, then the equipment list will be much larger and

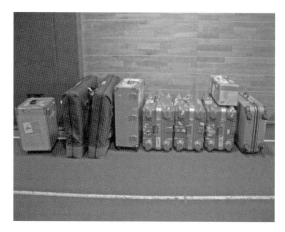

Figure 5.2 Medical and conditioning packages

commonly is the same equipment and supplies the team will take to the Olympics (see Chapter 6 for examples of equipment and supplies). In this case, the sports therapists must ensure there is sufficient supplies and equipment for both the training camp and the actual games (Figures 5.2, 5.3, and 5.4). Thus, it is essential that the sports therapist ensures he or she has appropriate and sufficient supplies, and that the equipment is in proper working order. In addition, the sport therapist must ensure that there are no custom restrictions or security issues related to any medical equipment or supplies that the team is bringing into the host country where the camp will be held and that he or she has

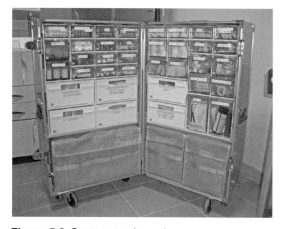

Figure 5.3 Custom-made package carry case

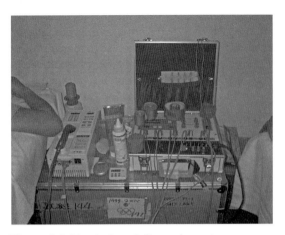

Figure 5.4 Physical modality equipment

appropriate power converters for the country so the equipment that is brought in can be used.

If each team of a delegation has a different training site, which is commonly the case, the sports therapist is often the only "medical" person accompanying the team and therefore commonly has a larger responsibility than just treating the injuries of the athlete. In effect, the sports therapist becomes the "medical team on site" and often has to deal with a number of issues that may not be directly related to the care and prevention of injuries such as nutrition, doping issues, psychological issues, issues outside his or her scope of practice, and personal interactions related to the athletes, coaches, and other support personnel, as well as medical issues commonly dealt with by a physician if he or she had been available. Thus, the role and responsibility of the sports therapist at training camps prior to a major games may be and often is much greater than his or her responsibilities during the actual games. To accomplish this enlarged role properly, the sports therapist must have a "team of advisors" available to communicate with in times of need. Thus, prior to traveling with a team, the sports therapist must develop this "team of medical advisors" whom he or she knows well and trusts and whom the therapist can call for advice on different issues which in some cases are beyond the normal scope of practice of the sports therapist.

Recently, several NOCs have tried to arrange a pre-event training camp for their whole Olympic team to enable the Olympic athletes to receive more systematic support, using a large facility near the Olympic venues. Such a pre-event camp, it is felt, enables the NOC to provide better care by enabling the athletes to have immediate access to their own physicians, sport therapists, nutritionists/dieticians, psychologists, and sport scientists, and helps to build team rapport and spirit. By having the training camp near the Olympic site, the athletes are given an opportunity to adapt to the environment of the site, local customs, and local foods. Such a venue also enables the information officer of the NOC to better provide timely information for the all athletes and coaches about the Olympic Games.

A pre-event training camp provides the sports therapist with an early opportunity to get to know the athletes and coaches he or she will be working with and to discover any conditions the athletes may have that are amenable to treatment. The presence of the sports therapist, in some cases with a physician, can prevent or decrease the severity of injuries and allow an early start to treatment of the injuries the athlete presently has. This may provide the athlete with an opportunity to recover while still training. In addition, the sports therapist, in collaboration with the physician, should have basic knowledge of doping and doping control so that he or she can ensure any medications or substances being taken by the athlete are within IOC regulations.

Preparation for the training camp

The selection of the place and facilities for the pre-event training camp involves a number of factors including a great deal of preparation. Such things as transportation, location of the training and conditioning facilities, and lodging and food services and security must be dealt with. Because of this, most athletes and coaches prefer a familiar place and facility that they have been to before rather than a new one. It is a big advantage to be familiar with the place and facility for the pre-event training camp as the team has a better understanding of the advantages and disadvantages of the site and the people involved before arriving, which decreases the stress level for everyone but especially the coaches and their athletes. Such a location will enhance the ability of the athlete to adapt to the training site more readily.

From a scientific point of view, sports therapists, if they are involved in the selection of a training site, have to ensure that the pre-event training camp is adequate to meet the needs of the athletes and coaches as well as the needs of the medical and support staff. Issues such as altitude, humidity, and temperature of the training site should, if possible, replicate these factors at the Olympic site. An exercise physiologist who is a specialist in high-altitude training might help the team monitor the adaptation of the athlete's physical condition if altitude is an issue at the Olympic competition site. Appropriate medical and conditioning facilities are also important in selecting a site. For example, the conditioning facility for recovery from extreme training or adaptation has to be prepared and equipped properly. Although the team commonly has several medical and conditioning individuals to help the athletes, it is important to include in the conditioning facilities such things as massage and therapy space, space for a pool and spa, and a re-fresh zone for effective conditioning support, along with access to a medical facility. Nutrition including appropriate food and drink (e.g., use of bottled water) is another concern as is ensuring appropriate sanitary conditions. Each athlete and team may have individual concerns that need to be dealt with to ensure the athletes can concentrate on their training with minimal distractions. Commonly, the sports therapist will work with team managers to ensure issues related to medical care and safety are dealt with.

Traveling to the training site/Olympic Games

Often, traveling to the pre-event training camp or site and/or the Olympic Games involves a long flight for athletes, coaches, and support staff. On the airplane, there is commonly lower atmospheric pressure and humidity compared with the ground

Table 5.1 Basic points to ensure proper hydration and to present venous thrombosis

To ensure proper hydration and to prevent venous thrombosis, the sports therapist should know the following basic points (Bartholomew *et al.* 2011):
1 Drink water or isotonic beverages to maintain adequate hydration
2 Exercise the legs at regular intervals
3 Walk around the cabin for 5 minutes on long flights (over 4 hours)
4 Avoid alcohol and caffeinated beverages, which are dehydrating
5 Avoid wearing tight clothing around the lower extremities and waist
6 Baggage should not be placed underneath the seat in front, as this reduces the ability to move the legs

level. This state can affect the athlete negatively. The atmospheric pressure on a flight is about 0.8 times ground level, which is the similar to an altitude of 1500 meters. The humidity on the flight is also low, often below 20% because of air conditioning. These conditions can lead to dehydration with increasing blood viscosity. In the worst case situations, these may cause pulmonary embolism and/or deep vein thrombosis. These potential effects will be even greater on long international flights. Thus, athletes should be encouraged, when appropriate, to move around the plane's cabin or do simple leg or foot exercise to stimulate circulation. Table 5.1 outlines some of the procedures the sport therapist should know.

A long flight commonly leads to jet lag and dehydration that can affect the circadian rhythms of the athletes and support personnel. In general, jet lag is greater on eastbound flights than on westbound flights. Recovery from westbound flights is 30–50% faster than eastbound flights. North–south flights cause minimal jet lag and have minimal effect on circadian rhythms. Support personnel including coaches and sport therapists must take this into account when considering initial training at the training site after flying long distances. It has been estimated that up to 1–3 days for each hour of time change is needed to adapt to the jet lag and to allow sleep patterns, heart rate, urinary output, and psychomotor performance to adjust. Younger people adapt more readily than older people. In order to minimize jet lag, individuals should depart well rested, with daylight departures (when traveling east, leave earlier; when traveling west, travel later), and the team should try to arrive at its destination close to bedtime. Eating and drinking should be moderate before and after flying and strenuous activity should be kept to a minimum in the first 24 hours after arrival.

Providing therapy services while traveling with a team

When traveling with a team and providing therapy services to the athlete, the sport therapist must be adaptable. With many sports, the sport therapist does more than just treat injuries. He or she must be prepared to "lend a hand" to make things for the athletes run as smoothly as possible. Thus, the sport therapist works closely with other support staff (especially the team manager) doing anything that is necessary to provide support to the athlete and coaches. When treating injuries, the sport therapist must also be adaptable and be able to provide services for the athlete anywhere, not just in a normal training room (Figure 5.5). The sport therapist must travel with all the supplies and equipment he or she will need so that time is not lost getting the proper equipment on site. The equipment and supplies needed will depend on the sport. Thus, the sport therapist must have good knowledge of the needs of the sports that he or she will be dealing with. One of the first things a sport therapist looks for at a new site is "where can I get ice?" to treat any recent injuries or to be prepared to treat any new injuries. It is the sports therapist's job to inspect any sleeping, eating, training, and competition sites to ensure the safety of the athletes under his or her care. He or she must find out about the emergency procedures used at training and competition sites and must be prepared to deal with any emergency situation involving team members, no matter how small.

Working with other health professionals "at a distance" or in different jurisdictions (e.g., traveling with a team when the therapist is the only support)

It is often important to collaborate with other health professionals to provide appropriate services to the athletes. This is especially true when each team has its individual training camp as opposed to a full Olympic team training camp. In these cases, it is common for the sport therapist to be the only "medical support" person available with the team. In this case, the sport therapist must find appropriate support in the local community, often relying

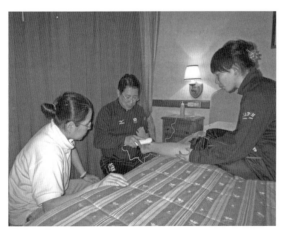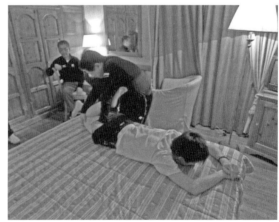

Figure 5.5 Therapy services at the lodging on training site

on local people for advice on whom to contact for different medical issues. Ideally, the team should have a local liaison/resource person who can help the team in times of need. In some cases, sport therapists have a "home country support team" whom he or she can call to ask advice on handling certain situations. Commonly, this may be the team physician who remains in the home country. In this case, there has to be very good rapport and trust between the physician and sport therapist.

How/who to seek information from regarding referrals, logistics, and supplies if traveling internationally with a team

If the sport therapist is going to travel internationally with the team, he or she must have proper personal up-to-date documentation (i.e., passport, visa) and the proper immunizations for the country or countries the team will be visiting. If possible, the sport therapist should contact the sport federation or the department of foreign affairs in his or her country for advice on the countries the team will be visiting and to ask the location and contact information of the embassy in the host country. If additional medical support is needed, it is a good idea to have the phone number of your country's embassy. By contacting the home embassy in the host country, the sport therapist can often find out, through the embassy, who the best medical staff are where the team is or at least whom the embassy staff use for medical care. Your country's embassy can be a great help, especially in times of serious need!

Commonly, sport therapists who travel with teams internationally have a great deal of experience at least locally or nationally with the sport with which they will be traveling. Thus, they will know the requirements of the sport in terms of medical needs. If they do not, they should contact the sport federation in their home country for the names of therapists who do know what the medical needs are and contact them for advice.

Traveling with an Olympic team prior to the Olympic Games for training camps and "friendly competitions" can be a rewarding and enjoyable experience for the sports therapist but also a stressful one. The sports therapist must be prepared to always *be available* 24/7 especially if he or she is the only medically related person with the team. The sports therapist must *be prepared* for anything by thinking of all the possible things that could affect the type of care for the athlete and support staff. If this is done before traveling, it will help relieve or prevent some of the stressful situations that are bound to occur during travel and training. The sports therapist should *be adaptable* as things do not always occur the way one hopes they will. Finally, the sports therapist must *be able to handle stressful situations* in a responsible way where the well-being of the athlete is the paramount concern. In these high pressure situations, such as the Olympics or prior to the Olympics, where the decisions made can affect athletes significantly (e.g., whether they are allowed to compete—something they have been training for years to do) can be a daunting task for any sports therapist.

Reference

Bartholomew, J.R., Schaffer, J.L. & McCormick, G.F. (2011) Air travel and venous thromboembolism: Minimizing the risk. *Cleveland Clinic Journal of Medicine*, 78(2), 111–120.

Chapter 6
Olympic event: logistical and treatment considerations

Nicola Phillips[1] and Caryl Becker[2]

[1] Cardiff University, Cardiff, UK
[2] British Olympic Association, London, UK

Background and typical role definition within an Olympic Games environment

Many countries' National Olympic Committees (NOC) that take part in an Olympic Games will recruit a physiotherapy support service pertinent to their individual needs, depending on team size and typical sport specificity of athletes registered for competition. Unfortunately, some countries may not be able to do this due to the size of their team and/or their ability to develop and provide the services of physiotherapists for their athletes. This chapter will concentrate on how countries should consider the development and provision of physiotherapy services for Olympic level athletes at the modern games. It is hoped that this guide will prove useful for those countries considering this.

Some NOCs will rely solely on the support facilities in the Olympic Village: at venues and at the polyclinics provided by the host country's organizing committee of the Olympic Games (OCOG) volunteer program, while others will aim to be self-sufficient regarding physiotherapy coverage. Some countries may strive for a balance between the two in order to capitalize on services available to meet the needs of their athletes.

For those NOCs aiming toward a self-sufficient physiotherapy support service, the number of phys-

iotherapists entering the village accredited as part of the NOC team (accredited physiotherapists) will vary considerably, depending on NOC or sport preferences, athlete numbers per sport, and number of accredited positions available. These accredited physiotherapists can either be selected and accredited directly through the NOC's allocation (NOC-accredited physiotherapists) or as happens in some NOCs, the sports themselves are offered a finite number of accreditations and the sport decides whether or not to accredit their physiotherapist (sport-specific physiotherapists). Utilizing a centralized NOC-provided physiotherapy service has the advantage of physiotherapists being able to be moved across sports as one sport finishes and another starts, thus maximizing the use of limited accreditations available for all officials of the countries delegation to the Olympics. The success of this will depend on the number of disciplines stated on a single accreditation pass, as it is this that allows the physiotherapist access to the accredited areas within the training and competition venues. There are a limited number of infinity passes available to any NOC as well as a limited number of passes that have up to three different disciplines stated—thereby allowing a physiotherapist to look after the athletes from three varying disciplines. The disadvantage of a centralized NOC physiotherapist system is that, for some sports, the

---

Sports Therapy Services, First Edition. Edited by James E. Zachazewski and David J. Magee.
© 2012 International Olympic Committee. Published 2012 by John Wiley & Sons, Ltd.

physiotherapist assigned by the NOC may not be the physiotherapist who has worked with the athletes in the period prior to the games.

Examples of different permutations on this concept are as follows:

1 Model A. A fully centralized NOC-provided service, with all physiotherapists traveling as part of the NOC central officials' accreditation allocation (centralized NOC accredited physiotherapists), then allocated to specific sport(s)/disciplines under one line management and covering each different sport when needed.

2 Model B. All physiotherapists are accredited from within the specific sport allocation(s) (sport-specific physiotherapists) and therefore only accredited for a single sport discipline, with no centralized service. Unfortunately, in this case, these physiotherapists are not able to assist with other sports or athletes who may need their services or expertise unless it is in the Olympic Village and the NOC's own accommodation. Use of accreditations in this manner may affect the number of accreditations available for coaches, team managers, or other personnel.

3 Model C. A mix of the above-mentioned points, with some sports prioritizing their officials' accreditations to one or more physiotherapists, plus an additional number of central NOC-provided physiotherapists who are able to cover a number of sports depending on areas of most need.

Table 6.1 outlines the impact on service provision depending on the mix of sport specific and NOC physiotherapists used. Much of the discussion in subsequent sections of this chapter centers around Model A and Model C, as Model B is coordinated solely through the sport. In addition, some sports will opt to take a nonaccredited physiotherapist, utilizing personal coach accreditations to access training venues but then require the centralized NOC or host OCOG volunteer support at the competition venue. The use of a "personal coach" accreditation in this way allows the sport/team to take physiotherapists who are more familiar with their athletes to support them during preparation for competition, and be able to use their accreditation allocation for other support staff such as more coaches or performance analysts who may be considered essential during competition for technical

or performance reasons. This scenario also relies on a centralized NOC physiotherapy service, housing sufficiently experienced physiotherapists who can adapt into this role, in any sport and with unfamiliar athletes, very quickly in order to provide continuity of care.

Planning—prior to departure

Some of the planning can be done ahead of time based on electronic information available, such as practice and competition schedules. Other information can be gathered by the head physiotherapist if he or she is included as part of the "reconnaissance team" visits to the host city by the NOC medical staff. A physiotherapist with previous elite/international experience can be an invaluable member of the planning process. Planning is critical between the head physiotherapist and other members of the NOC's medical staff.

Service prioritization for recruitment

Even at the very early stages of preparation, prioritizing which services will be provided within a NOC's physiotherapy team is important for recruitment and planning. This prioritization will largely depend on numbers of athletes qualified and preference of specific sports. This helps directly the makeup of the medical and physiotherapy support team for the competition. Criteria for recruitment usually prioritizes skills and experience that complement the identified needs of the NOC and teams competing. Central NOC appointments tend to be better suited for those physiotherapists who have sufficient experience at an elite Olympic level as they are better able to transfer skills across sports, sometimes at short notice if covering illnesses or unanticipated additional workload. Central NOC physiotherapy staff require multiple skills to cover both performance-related soft tissue work and injury assessment and management. Typical criteria for these individuals can be seen in Table 6.2.

Once selected as part of the centralized NOC physiotherapy staff, part of the performance

Table 6.1 Impact on service provision depending on the mix of sport-specific and NOC physiotherapists used

	Sport-Specific Physiotherapist (Accredited to a Single Sports Venue Training and Competition)	Sport-Specific Physiotherapist (Nonaccredited)	NOC Physiotherapist (Accredited for all Training/Competition Venues)
Training venue	*Full* access	*Limited* access if personal coach accreditation used	*Full* access to specific sport venues
	Could utilize NOC physiotherapists as additional cover for busy periods given different logistics of a multisport games	Could utilize NOC physiotherapy cover depending on risk assessment/numbers	
	Complete continuity of care	*Compromised* continuity of care	*Compromised* continuity of care unless able to get to know sport and athletes before start of the games
Competition venue	*Full* access	*No* access	*Full* access to specific sport venues
		NOC physiotherapist with full access would cover venue	NOC would cover all venues
	Complete continuity of care	*Compromised* continuity of care	*Compromised* continuity of care unless familiarization period used prior to the games. Complete continuity between training and competition periods
Performance center (OLV)	*Full* access until the end of their sports competition schedule	Access *limited* to between 9 AM and 9 PM on prearranged "day pass"	*Full* access at all times
	Able to use additional support from NOC staff for specialist input for specific or complex injuries if needed.	Able to get additional support from NOC for specialist input for specific or complex injuries if needed.	Provide specialist skills to add value where requested
	Able to access NOC staff for additional support such as massage	Able to access NOC staff for additional support such as massage	
	Complete continuity of care	*Complete* continuity of care if able to get in every day on a day pass.	*Compromised* continuity but added value and additional support
		Compromised if treatment required before 9 AM or after 9 PM	
Other	Able to work continually with the athletes in the lead up to the games	Able to work continually with the athletes in the lead up to the games	Variable capacity to work with the athletes in the lead up to the games.

management process would be to agree on set objectives that the individual physiotherapists might hope to achieve as part of their responsibilities to the team and for their personal development.

Specifics regarding this process and its benefits are detailed later in this chapter. After selection for the games, any training requirements would be covered as part of an orientation to the NOC

Table 6.2 Typical criteria based recruitment of NOC physiotherapy support team

Clinical Skills and Experience Requirements	Preferred Behavioral Characteristics
• Competencies equivalent of International Federation of Sports Physical Therapy (IFSPT) accredited sports physiotherapist www.ifspt.org • Min 1 multisport games, such as Commonwealth, Pan-American, Asian or World University or Youth Olympic Games (typical on an NOC team would be experience of at least four of these opportunities) • Postgraduate sports massage qualifications as part of sports specialization route • Evidence of ongoing commitment to high-performance sport • Current advanced sports trauma management certificate	• Calm under pressure • Conscious awareness of skill level and team mechanics • Focus on performance target • Good personal organization and time keeping • Ability to perform by adapting to different sporting environments • Experienced and knowledgeable • Interpersonal skills and communication: A team player

physiotherapy staff. Often times, these relate to record keeping systems, maintaining adequate treatment statistics for reporting following the games period, and expected professional behaviors and values to consider as staff representing their country.

Coordinating services with sports-specific physiotherapy staff

A significant amount of workforce planning will center around the practice and competition schedule, which will drive the physiotherapy support requirements on a daily basis. Although this only provides a basic overview until final athlete selection is confirmed, it can form the basis of logistics for allocating NOC-provided physiotherapists to sports. Early allocation is desired to allow familiarization of physiotherapists with the sport and the individual athletes competing, if these individuals (the physiotherapist and the team) have not been working together prior to the games.

Responsibilities of the physiotherapy leader would include investigating professional licensure and practice issues, indemnity insurance, and any restrictions to practice specific to the host country prior to departure. In some countries, an application has to be made for a temporary license to practice during the games period. In all cases, the physiotherapists are usually restricted to treating members of their NOC team only and would not be ensured to treat athletes or officials from other countries. Some countries have differing restrictions on whether specific treatment modalities or equipment are covered under the national legislation.

Managing expectations based on accreditation and access limitations

Accreditations allocated for officials (Ao accreditations) for each NOC will be calculated using IOC Rule 39 and is based on, amongst others, athlete numbers qualified for each sport, with differing permutations for team and individual sports. Therefore, sports that qualify a small number of athletes may not reach the required numbers to trigger sufficient Ao accreditations for a team manager, coach(es) *plus* medical/physiotherapy staff coverage. Other sports with specific technical or performance needs may have to prioritize their allocation to more technical coaches, performance analysts, psychologists, or to other types of staff required to support the athlete achieving their highest level of performance at the Olympic event. These sports will be more likely to require that physiotherapy support be provided by the centralized NOC physiotherapy team.

Other team sports such as hockey, football, basketball, or others may accredit one physiotherapist but request additional support for busy periods from the centralized service as backup personnel. For example, sports such as swimming may manage quite well with their sports-specific allocation for the majority of the games period but request help for relay days when larger numbers of competitors require support for recovery between heats and finals. This is typically supported via the centralized NOC support service in a combined setup, such as is described in Table 6.1.

It is important that team managers, coaches, and athletes are all aware of the chosen physiotherapy support delivery system so that expectations of the type and amount of coverage available during the games, as well as identifying who the individuals are and who will be delivering the service, are understood well ahead of time. This allows for the development of appropriate strategies to manage all physiotherapy needs for competition time.

Travel

Flight bookings and other travel arrangements have to be put in place well ahead of the games period. Any travel grants or sponsored travel usually requires early bookings. Decisions have to be made about any advance party numbers needed to set up the clinic and liaise with the OCOG volunteer medical personnel at the polyclinic and the various venues prior to the official Olympic Village opening. Therefore, accommodation for those first few days before accredited staff are allowed to stay in the Olympic Village overnight will also have to be booked. This "soft opening," which is a few days prior to the official opening of the Olympic Village and the arrival of the NOC staff, allows for logistics and setup needs to be accomplished in an efficient manner prior to any athletes arriving into the Olympic Village. Physiotherapy arrivals into the Olympic Village are ideally planned according to the estimated numbers needed for unpacking and setting up the NOC's own treatment clinic/area and anticipated athlete arrivals, which will be more or less staggered, depending on whether pre-Olympic training camps are used.

Planning amount, type, and freight of equipment

Planning the required amount of equipment needed to deliver the services required by all

athletes and consumable products, such as tape or massage lotion, can be a challenge. This is particularly so when the competition sites are geographically distant so that sufficient freight time is allowed to transport equipment and supplies. If sea freight is used, rather than air freight, the equipment and consumables are likely to be shipped before final team numbers are known, especially in events where selection is late. Table 6.3 provides a list of typical physiotherapy equipment and consumable supplies required for a team of 200–300 athletes. A few of the challenging questions and concerns that the head physiotherapist and team planners must consider at the planning stage are described as follows:

How much tape should be ordered for a team of 200–300 athletes? This is particularly challenging if the spread of potential numbers includes unknown numbers of sports that would typically be heavy users of consumables, for examples, field sports and team sports. There may also be restrictions for different sports regarding color or type of tape, for example, gymnastics, where only flesh colored tape is allowed.

How much massage medium should be ordered? What are athlete preferences for oil versus lotion across different sports? There may also be restrictions for different sports regarding use of either medium related to performance, for example, water polo or weightlifting prohibiting use of oil.

How many treatment bed/tables will be needed? Planning for this should take into account the number and type of beds/tables supplied by the host country, as well as the number an NOC may order from the "rate card." The "rate card" being a list of equipment put together by the organizing committee from which an NOC can rent items for the duration of the games. This list can incorporate anything from additional chairs to electrotherapy machines. These beds/tables would typically be nonadjustable treatment couches. NOC clinic space, venue requirements, numbers of athletes, and numbers of physiotherapists would all factor into estimation of requirement.

How many sports will be planning on using ice recovery strategies in the Games Village clinic? Is ice available? How difficult is it to get? Ice in sufficient quantity is often times difficult to get in many

Table 6.3 Typical physiotherapy equipment and consumable supplies required for a team of 200–300 athletes

Item	Approximate Quantity	Comments
Dressings (various)	100s	Sufficient for different size and types of wounds and enough for distribution amongst venue bags
Tape (rigid various widths)	200 rolls	As/above
Tape (elastic adhesive various widths)	150 rolls	As/above
Felt/Padding/Fleecy web	50 sheets	As/above
Tubular bandage	1 box of each size	As/above
Cohesive bandage (various sizes and types)	90 rolls	As/above
Ankle/knee/wrist/thigh braces	At least one of each size and side	
Wound management sprays (various types)	20+[a]	Sufficient for different size and types of wounds and enough for distribution amongst venue bags
Sterile saline sachets/pods	75–100	
Various creams/powders (insect bites/minor skin irritations, etc.)	50[a]	
Smelling salts	[a]	
Antiseptic wipes	150	
Massage lotion/cream	6–7 L	
Massage oil	5–6 L	
Pre-tape spray	[a]	
Acupuncture needles (various sizes)	250	
Tape cutters/scissors	[a]	
Tweezers	[a]	
Fixation straps	[a]	
Exercise band/tubing	1 pack of each strength/color	
Ice wrap/ice bags		
Sharps disposal boxes	2	
Cotton buds	100	
Disposable razors		
Latex and nonlatex gloves	200	
Ultrasound gel		
Electrotherapy/ultrasound equipment	3/4	
Portable/adjustable treatment beds	22	These numbers will depend on the number of sites to be covered, across venues and possible satellite Games Villages
Crutches	3 pairs	
Portable ice recovery baths	2/3	

[a]Denotes numbers of items needed for each venue kit bag, which will depend on physiotherapist numbers as well as athlete requirements.

countries around the world. The number of sports requesting ice recovery support will significantly affect the amount of ice needed on a daily basis, which will have to be factored into provision. Consideration also has to be given to how many portable ice recovery baths to freight out depending on whether some sports bring their own equipment. How the ice is to be transported around the village is also important—is there a need for a large cooler box on wheels and smaller cooler boxes that allow transport of ice to a venue? If so, these would be transported with the freight.

Will the chosen freight transport involve extremes of temperature? Different adhesive tape or rubberized items do not travel well in extremes of heat. Therefore, temperature-controlled containers may be required to ensure that the equipment is usable on arrival.

Are there any customs regulations, flight carrier restrictions, or security consideration in the destination country regarding equipment freighted? Different countries and their national airlines will have different regulations and some will vary depending on mode of transport for freight. This could affect some of the type of consumable supplies the NOC plans on using. For instance, some countries will not allow air freight of any aerosols without a specific license that needs to be purchased in advance. Others may not allow specific products into the country. Customs regulations and the time taken to clear customs will also vary and therefore freight planning has to allow for potential delays. Additional time may also be needed to allow Games Village security, which would be over and above national customs regulations, to inspect and clear supplies. This can sometimes take a few days to a week for large consignments. This may be especially true with equipment that might contain restricted substances and items such as sharp implements.

Other equipment may not be suitable for freighting. One example is industrial sized ice machines. They may have to be ordered on the host city organizers' rate card. Estimating the amount of ice production required will rely on communication with sports regarding their planned use of any ice recovery strategies for performance, as this will significantly increase the ice required over and above that needed for injury management. As ice recovery is often done in the same area of the NOC clinic/treatment area, it is usually the physiotherapy team who manages recovery as well as injury management to maximize use of available accreditations.

Information gathering visit

Some NOCs will send all team managers for each sport plus the NOC management team, including physiotherapy, on a "reconnaissance visit." This usually happens close enough to the Games Village opening date but prior to security lockdown of village and venues. Such a visit allows familiarization with likely travel times between venues. From a visit such as this, a more detailed plan for competition coverage can be developed, the optimal physical layout of rooms determined, and a plan for how the clinic/treatment area will be set up can be completed. This is also the time when small details such as numbers and types of electrical sockets, the need for extension cords, power converters, and the need for a specific number of Internet connections required in the clinic/treatment area within the Games Village are determined; development of emergency access plans and facilities for field of play at training and competition venues are completed; visits to the hospitals involved with the games are completed; and, if appropriate, meetings held with key host city management staff. Preparations for workforce planning within the team can then be modified before final team departure if necessary.

Planning any further items that may be needed and obtained through the usual "rate card" system may also be discussed and modified at this time, depending on space and distance from various athlete services provision within the Games Village.

Communication

Communication within the physiotherapy team will be important to plan for various incidents that would require changes in plans on a day-to-day basis. Appropriate provision for temporary mobile phones or SIM cards that can be inserted into existing mobile phones should be considered. These phones would usually be purchased by the general management of the NOC. Numbers needed and accessibility requirements would be determined by the lead physiotherapist during the planning stage. Communication links for different emergencies would be planned within the physiotherapy and medical staff as well as with team management at this stage. It is critical that a communication cascade be prearranged and disseminated, using mobile phones, or Blackberries[TM], depending on the assessed telecommunications challenges of a specific country before arrival on site.

Prior to Departure Checklist

Liaise with NOC management and sports regarding physiotherapy team size and potential HQ/sports-specific mix	✓
Set and implement recruitment criteria	✓
Investigate license to practice, indemnity insurance, and legal therapeutic use restrictions issues specific to host country	✓
Liaise with sports on likely requests for support depending on sport-specific numbers and identified busy periods	✓
Identify departure times for physiotherapists to coincide with preparation needs and athlete arrivals	✓
Estimate/order equipment and consumables quantities based on smallest/largest time size scenarios	✓
Identify and plan around freight logistics for protection of equipment and legislative regulations	✓
Order/pack physiotherapy equipment/consumables	✓
Order any large items to be hired from the rate card system	✓
Information from reconnaissance visit used to modify existing plans	✓
Within team communication channels planned—i.e., mobile phones or Blackberries. Local SIM card availability	✓
Identify and deliver any staff training required prior to departure (such as record keeping treatment statistics process)	✓

Planning—on arrival

Unpacking, stock check, and clinic setup

Much of this work is typically quite physical and may take time and effort of many of the physiotherapy team. For a team of 200–300 athletes, three physiotherapists would typically be required/scheduled to start the initial setup at "soft opening" of the Olympic Village site. One or two more of the staff would arrive a few days to a week later to help with further stock management and setup.

A clinic/treatment area is usually set up in the athletes' village or accommodation area. This often means converting a flat or apartment into a clinic, as illustrated in Figure 6.1. It also involves arranging communal and private treatment spaces, office areas for record keeping with all the necessary electronic and Internet systems available. Secure storage space is required if paper-based note keeping is used, as well as general storage space for equipment and consumables.

This is also the time when "rate card" items are procured and installed in appropriate spaces. For instance, ice machines may need to be installed in shower areas or bathrooms to make use of existing plumbing arrangement as substantial changes to apartments are usually very limited, as they would typically be sold following the games period. A television may seem a luxury item but using one installed in the clinic area is often the way physiotherapists see most of the games. Knowing whether an athlete has performed well or not, through a television in the clinic, is extremely valuable to be able to anticipate likely athlete behavior, in order to modify the treatment environment accordingly, for the benefit of that athlete and others around them.

Volunteer domestic services provision

Services such as laundry of towels or any other necessary linen need to be negotiated at this stage. Towels in the numbers required by physiotherapists to minimize cross infection is often underestimated by Games Village services. Similarly, the load on laundry services for this aspect can be significant. Different host services and countries will have varying provision for this, with some regarding towels used for massage as clinically soiled and others as regular laundry. Liaising with the appropriate vendor, service, or volunteer sector for this is important to clarify before the clinic starts getting busy. Agreeing about times when it is appropriate to clean the clinic area and the level of cleaning also needs communicating at an early stage. It should be

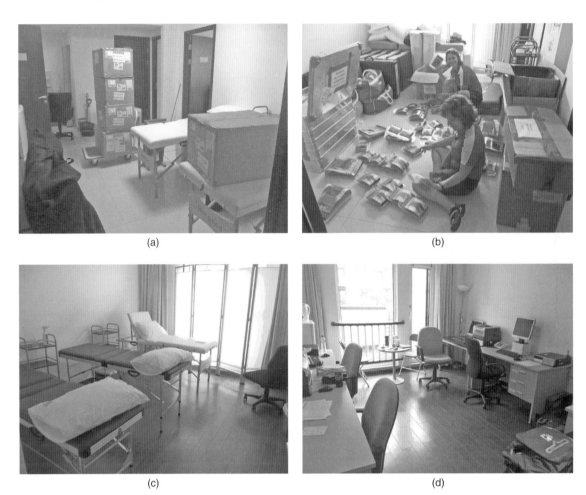

(a)

(b)

(c)

(d)

Figure 6.1 Setting up clinic/treatment area (a) equipment and stock is delivered to an accommodation block (b) unpacking and stock checking (c) typical set up of a bedroom converted to a clinical area (d) typical set up of a bedroom converted to an office area for record keeping and clinically related administrative work

remembered that this is a clinical health care area and acceptable standards of cleanliness are greater than for general living accommodation.

Check each venue and meet emergency personnel

On arrival, physiotherapists would also use this time to visit the key venues they would be covering to check facilities. Close attention should be paid to which exit is to be used for emergencies, which hospital that the injured athletes will be taken to, drive times, and phone numbers for hospitals and emer-

gency transports services. Also, typical routes between warm-up and competition areas, opportune places that could be used for last minute treatment that might be required, and any accreditation-related access limitations that could affect communication are also checked. These lighter tasks are often good use of "acclimatization time." Just as the competing athlete needs to recover from a long-haul flight and possible time zone changes, the physiotherapist also requires that same time and consideration to maintain a high level of clinical performance throughout the games period.

Negotiating field of play access in emergencies can be a sensitive issue and will change from sport to sport. If field of play access is strictly limited to host city provision, then an area where team physiotherapists are able to meet with their athletes should be identified prior to athlete arrival so that arrangements can be communicated with the team manager beforehand to avoid confusion in the event of any problems during competition. In the case of an emergency, all personnel can manage the injured athlete efficiently and effectively.

On Arrival Checklist

Stock unpacked and checked for any missing items	✓
Ice machines, television, computer, Internet points installed	✓
Treatment beds unpacked and set up, signs to assist finding the clinic, communication boards to inform athletes of physiotherapists' location	✓
Clinic laundry and cleaning provision clarified and agreed	✓
Venue emergency procedures and exits ascertained	✓
Any communication black-spots at venues identified	✓
Field of play and link area access limitations identified	✓
Distances between accommodation block/clinic and dining areas, transport mall, polyclinic, laundry	✓

Communication between team medical professionals and host country and team officials

Communication is a critical factor between NOC physiotherapists and the rest of the medical team as well as between host city/OCOG volunteer officials. Before athletes' arrival, physiotherapists should check that there is mobile telecommunication signal/access in various areas of venues. Since warm-up and treatment sectors are often underneath large buildings, areas where there is limited reception is not uncommon. Testing this beforehand ensures that in the case of an emergency, the physiotherapist would know where to go to contact the team

physiotherapists and medical staff covering back in the Games Village if assistance or additional cover is needed urgently.

Prioritizing service provision

Once athletes arrive in the Games Village, the work starts to resemble a more typical sports physiotherapy role involving athlete management. With the inevitable restrictions of physiotherapy accreditations based on athlete numbers, there will always be an element of prioritization of care, whichever of the staffing and coverage options highlighted in the earlier section are used. Considerations are given to issues such as the following:

- **Sports-Specific Injury Risk.** As a general principle, the sports included within each Olympic Games can be broadly categorized into groups for prioritizing need, based on likely injury incidence and/or severity. For example, contact/collision sports and field sports such as football, hockey, basketball, and rugby 7s would be regarded as high-risk sports. Individual sports such as gymnastics, equestrian, or diving would also fit into this category, as an injury sustained in these sports would statistically have more chance of being of a serious nature. Alternatively, while injuries are also sustained in sports such as shooting or archery, they are less likely to be life threatening. Some sports also have mandatory medical/physiotherapy support as part of their regulations, such as boxing, judo, rugby, and taekwondo.

- **Highlighted Ongoing Injury/Recovery Issues for Any Individual Athlete in a Sport.** Despite, what could be the best support and preparation in the lead up to an Olympic Games, there can be instances where athletes are still caring for minor injuries, which still allows them to compete to their full potential with appropriate help. The athlete may also have a known history of illness that might require support at the competition site in case of emergency, such as asthma, diabetes, or epilepsy. The preference in these instances would be to prioritize NOC medical cover, but on occasions, the limitations within a team means that this role could well be coordinated by a physiotherapist who would brief the OCOG venue medical support in an emergency.

• **Competition versus Training Coverage.** Many sports have a subdivision of events or competitions, for gender, weight categories, disciplines, or events. This means that there is likely to be a diverse training and competition schedule planned within the sport, with some athletes remaining in the Games Village, some training and some competing at any one time. Physiotherapy coverage has to be prioritized and this is often where a combined approach, using centralized NOC support, is most useful. Careful planning is needed to provide physiotherapy resources to an athlete working through a daily schedule for an evening competition, while also covering a training session or competition at the other end of the day. For many of the individual sports, some athletes will still be training on days when their teammates are competing. In these instances, priority would usually be given to those competing, with secondary support from either physiotherapy colleagues within the NOC support team or host city OCOG provision for the others.

However, in some cases, the physiotherapist's role might be perceived as more valuable to be based in the Olympic Village during the competition than at the venue site. This might be the case in sports such as cycling or skiing, where the nature of the event means that access during competition might be limited relative to where an injury might occur, or if an injury does occur, it is often likely to be serious enough to require immediate medical management and transfer back to the Olympic Village or to a hospital, with no prospect of continuing in that specific competition.

• **Performance Potential of the Individual or Team.** Prioritizing an individual or team that is in the running for a medal is considered but should not be at the expense of the risk factors detailed earlier. The athlete's welfare is always the highest priority for any health care personnel who has a duty of care toward that athlete. However, an athlete who is a medal potential may need to be prioritized as they are often more likely to compete longer through the event, such as through heats to finals. Similarly, a medal winning team will usually have competed through early rounds then knockout matches over a 2-week period and again may require prioritizing due to the risk of overuse-type injuries.

• **Transportation and Distance to and from the Venue.** If it has been ascertained that covering a specific sport is a priority, the distance of the venue from the Olympic Village can have a significant impact on the ability of the physiotherapist to cover that event in addition to anything else, such as a second event or a clinic session in the Games Village. Some competition sites could be up to an hour's journey each way, which does not allow help to be sent on request in case of need. Other venues are likely to be closer but could still be a few miles apart from each other. Usually, all athlete transportation goes via the Olympic Village as a hub and not between venues. Therefore, unless a team car is made available, physiotherapists covering across venues would need to go back to the Olympic Village and back out again, increasing traveling times. This again assumes that the physiotherapist's accreditation allows access into more than the one or three venues stated on their accreditation pass.

Prioritization of Service Provision Checklist

Modified risk analysis of sports on arrival	✓
Any ongoing injury highlighted	✓
Training and competition plans received from sports	✓
Any additional cover requirements highlighted, based on changing demands	✓
Potential individuals requiring greater support identified	✓
Reporting back any issues related to venue transport that might affect timing of cover	✓

Logistics

The logistics of day-to-day running of the physiotherapy service will be shaped by the constraints of staffing available and the prioritized factors previously highlighted. Organization can be complex and liable to be changeable at short notice, requiring a high degree of flexibility within the system to be able to adapt to competing needs. Factors affecting decision making for this element will include location of the event, travel times, specific skills needed, and staffing needed at specific times, as well as regulations of the sport.

Day-to-Day Logistics Checklist

Daily planner sheet populated with physiotherapist schedule for the following day	✓
Individual athlete competition support requirements identified and rehearsed if necessary	✓
Contemporaneous treatment records completed to ensure that any treatment handover is accurate	✓
Any emergency communication cascade available to the NOC staff covering the clinic	✓
Transport timetables to all venues available in the clinic	✓
Any messages from sports-specific physiotherapists identified and actioned on a daily basis	✓

Precompetition period following official opening

The competition schedule of an Olympic Games means that sports could start any time from a few days before the opening ceremony, as in the case of football, the following day, or any time in the remaining 2-week period. Athletes usually arrive with their sport any time from a week to a few days prior to their event, depending on whether their NOC has opted to use a pre-Olympic preparation camp. Once athletes arrive in the Olympic Village, training days are a very useful opportunity to establish a rapport if the NOC physiotherapist has only had limited access to these athletes prior to the games, compared with the sports-specific physiotherapists. This is particularly relevant if the NOC-accredited physiotherapist is likely to be acting as an extra pair of hands at busy times. It is important that athletes become familiar with any physiotherapists who are new to the team if they are to be involved in any way during training or competition. As described earlier, NOC-nominated physiotherapists who are

supporting sports with smaller numbers would usually have already started establishing this relationship prior to the team's departure, once the decision to use NOC physiotherapy provision had been confirmed.

Sometimes, a sport realizes that their planned sport-specific physiotherapist may not be able to work as well as planned due to accreditation access. In this case, NOC physiotherapist staff will often need to be assigned to a team or sport. This pre-games period can then be used to problem-solve and allow NOC physiotherapy staff to become acquainted with the athletes of that team or sport.

During competition period

Managing service provision on a day-to-day basis

Figure 6.2 describes a typical daily planning sheet for physiotherapy support across 10 members of staff. Sports are arbitrary examples, but the pattern is typical of work at the busiest period during games time, with very little rest opportunity. Although clinic times are included as 7:30 AM–10:30 PM, these are guidelines and the asterisks represent the areas that required cover either before 7:30 AM start or after 10:30 PM finish that day. Planning also requires consideration of maintaining resilience of staff and, therefore, even during the busiest times, timetabling a slightly later start or earlier finish when possible is important to ensure a quality service through the end of the games period. These clinic times and venue cover also need to include time for record keeping, which is a professional mandatory requirement linked to license to practice in most countries, as well as being a means of collecting vital information for future workforce planning. There will be national variation in amount and type of record keeping as well as the use of electronic or hard copy systems. Whichever method is used needs to provide accessible information for review, while being sufficiently secure for individual patient confidentiality.

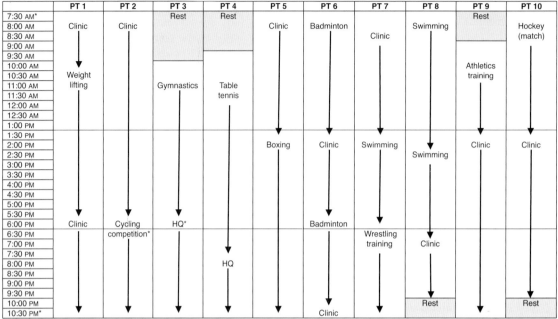

	PT 1	PT 2	PT 3	PT 4	PT 5	PT 6	PT 7	PT 8	PT 9	PT 10
7:30 AM*	Clinic	Clinic	Rest	Rest	Clinic	Badminton		Swimming	Rest	Hockey
8:00 AM							Clinic			(match)
8:30 AM										
9:00 AM										
9:30 AM										
10:00 AM	Weight								Athletics	
10:30 AM	lifting								training	
11:00 AM			Gymnastics	Table						
11:30 AM				tennis						
12:00 AM										
12:30 AM										
1:00 PM										
1:30 PM										
2:00 PM					Boxing	Clinic	Swimming		Clinic	Clinic
2:30 PM								Swimming		
3:00 PM										
3:30 PM										
4:00 PM										
4:30 PM										
5:00 PM										
5:30 PM										
6:00 PM	Clinic	Cycling	HQ*			Badminton				
6:30 PM		competition*					Wrestling	Clinic		
7:00 PM							training			
7:30 PM										
8:00 PM				HQ						
8:30 PM										
9:00 PM										
9:30 PM										
10:00 PM								Rest		Rest
10:30 PM*						Clinic				

*Guideline times which change depending on specific demand.

Figure 6.2 Typical daily planning sheet for physiotherapy support

Venue coverage

Covering both competition and training venues as well as the clinic within the NOC setup can be challenging, given the accreditation limitations, as previously explained. Therefore, prioritization of what becomes essential and can only be successful if there is excellent communication. In some sports, the training venue is on the same site as the competition venue, which allows the covering physiotherapist to move between both areas dependent on the competition and training schedules. Other sports use entirely different sites for training, which increases the logistical difficulty of covering both areas once competition has started. Therefore, some difficult decisions sometimes have to be made. Good communication with athletes, often via the team managers, allows planning to cover specific times, when the athlete has identified that they require physiotherapy support, without necessarily having to be present for the whole training or competition session. If a physiotherapist has to move between sites, the success of this strategy also relies on a good athlete transport system or sufficient advance notice to request use of a team vehicle, which would be assessed on a needs basis.

NOC clinic cover for recovery/injury management

Contact patterns in the NOC clinic/treatment area generally fall into two categories, namely, injury and performance related.

1 Injury. Often the injuries seen in the NOC clinic are a secondary assessment, with the athlete having been assessed at the training or competition venue when the injury occurred. Depending on the severity of the problem, further investigation might be required in conjunction with the medical team, possibly using OCOG polyclinic imaging facilities. Other more minor injuries would be managed within the clinic following possible immediate management at the venue if it was deemed appropriate. In these instances, further management of the injury during competition would be discussed and, if necessary, rehearsed for timing and within confines of available treatment opportunities available during competition. For example, a weightlifter may require a specific soft tissue technique between lifts, when there is a very strict time restriction. Therefore, any modification to a technique to allow adapted positioning would need to be practiced and timed before attempting use in a competition setting.

2 Performance. A large proportion of the workload while covering the NOC clinic is likely to be performance based, particularly involving recovery. For example, if there is a physiotherapy lead for a specific sport, regardless of whether he or she is accredited through the sport or the NOC physiotherapy support allocation, that practitioner assumes the lead on managing the athletes injury when present, with a second or sometimes even a third physiotherapist providing additional help. This typically resembles a pattern of the lead physiotherapist assessing and treating any newly reported injuries, while the supporting physiotherapists provided recovery support. Recovery support may take the form of massage, ice baths, or some other type of intervention. However, it is rarely as simple in reality, with a major proportion of the massage contacts involving some form of physiotherapy intervention alongside the pure recovery work. Communication between physiotherapists during these times is essential to ensure best practice as well as avoiding potentially overtreating through duplication.

Venues coverage and manning NOC clinic in the village

The points above illustrate the importance of providing coverage at both sites. Creating an ideal balance between the two is a challenge. Because of the potentially reactive nature of work in the NOC clinic, in addition to recovery support, there always has to be a member of staff present to deal with any urgent unanticipated treatment requests. Also, in the event of an emergency, the staff within the clinic need to coordinate communication and amend coverage between other members of the team if the physiotherapist covering the venue had to accompany an athlete to the emergency treatment area of the polyclinic or to a designated emer-

gency hospital. Figure 6.3 illustrates an example of a typical process for injury management and communication between venue and village support.

Liaising with sports-specific physiotherapists for when they need help

The competition schedule will highlight some areas of anticipated high demand for physiotherapy support well in advance. In addition, as competition progresses, other areas of high demand will become apparent if athletes are successful in the early stages. Good liaison between central NOC physiotherapists and sport-specific staff will facilitate planning for any additional cover needed for these later stages of competition. Conversely, other sports may well need less cover as the competition progresses and therefore workforce planning can be adapted to the changing circumstances during the games period.

Covering venues where there is no sports-specific cover

Where staffing is limited, prioritization is based on the criteria discussed earlier. Wherever possible, the NOC physiotherapist would travel to the competition venue with the competing athletes and be at hand for any support needed during preparation and competition. Support may also be needed immediately postcompetition, which could be particularly important if the athlete is either competing in subsequent rounds or further events. In this instance, the NOC physiotherapist functions in exactly the same way as a sports-specific physiotherapist.

Responding to changing circumstances

Occasionally, a sports-specific physiotherapist becomes ill or gets injured and is therefore unable to provide the planned support. Although infrequent, at least one incidence is likely to occur in a reasonable sized team. A physiotherapist with any infection such as an upper respiratory tract infection is at risk of spreading illness to athletes and would

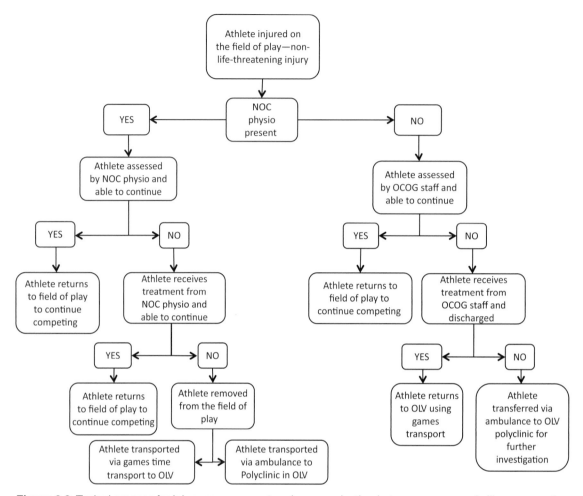

Figure 6.3 Typical process for injury management and communication between venue and village support

usually be isolated until he or she is no longer infectious. During this time, a physiotherapist from the centralized NOC team would undertake to cover that support and this would require further flexibility in the system as well as individuals with the skills and experience to instill confidence at short notice.

Concluding stages

Packing up

Everything tends to happen very quickly at the end of the games and there is the temptation to try

and get a head start by packing up before all athletes have finished competing. Although doing this takes some of the pressure off the physiotherapy team, it is important to ensure that athletes still competing on the final day enter a clinic that is fully functional with no evidence of any diminution of service. Any packing up that is done should leave the clinic looking, at face value, as if nothing has changed.

Stocktaking all consumables before packing them up takes time but can be invaluable in informing future lead physiotherapists about the amount of consumables used and therefore what needs to be ordered next time around. All boxes have to be labeled with contents lists and appropriate destination addresses for customs and freight purposes. If labeled appropriately, the process will also avoid more work once home. Some stock has a shelf life that could expire prior to the next Olympic Games and would therefore need to be used during the following cycle, whereas other stock will be ongoing supplies for storage. Identifying items in this is useful to prevent wastage and maintain supplies of possibly more expensive items used minimally but needed for specific instances.

Deciding who flies back with the team and who stays behind to pack and clean can also be an important decision as it is always advisable to have someone from the medical team on the flight home with the athletes. The rest of the physiotherapy team may need to stay over for a day or two to pack up and help the NOC with all the finalities involved with leaving the village. This will include someone from the organizing committee checking all the equipment ordered through the "rate card."

Finally, it may prove worthwhile to consider taking a few days annual leave before returning to one's normal place of work. This allows one not only to relax and recover but also to synthesize all that has happened during 4 weeks of an Olympic Games.

Concluding Stages Checklist

Equipment and remaining stock itemized, packed, and labeled for freight departure, including all necessary customs paperwork	✓
All rate card items returned and accounted for to prevent any additional payments	✓
All staff flights confirmed and ensuring at least one member of the medical team travels with the main athlete return flight	✓
Follow-up performance reviews arranged for a date after returning home	✓
Debrief report compiled using treatment statistics and including recommendations for future games	✓

Staff appraisal

As part of the performance management of staff, each physiotherapist should complete a self-appraisal form before departure, highlighting what they aimed to achieve during the period of the Olympic Games, both in terms of athlete support and their own personal and professional development. Figure 6.4 illustrates a typical template form for objective planning and reflection.

Following the games, a debrief meeting is planned on an individual basis between the lead physiotherapist and each individual physiotherapist in the team. If the physiotherapy support is not organized through the NOC, this should be done through the individual sports' National Governing Bodies, who are usually the physiotherapist's employer. The meeting should ideally take place soon enough after the games for the discussion to be relevant but leaving enough time to recover and reflect. However, as this means a separate meeting on return to the home country, it may not be practicable and should then be done at a mutually convenient time.

Following up a busy Olympic Games work period in this way can seem a lot of effort, but the process is invaluable for succession management through development of appropriate skills and attitudes of the support teams behind the athletes.

Figure 6.5 describes the type of questions used to guide the reflection and appraisal related to behavior and performance.

Debrief report

Within a few months of returning after an Olympic Games, there is usually a debrief meeting, containing reports from key work areas. This would include a physiotherapy report. Content of the report should include details of all areas discussed in the sections above, highlighting areas that worked well and those that did not, with recommendations of good practice which could be used in future, as well as suggestions for improvement. Information also needs to be provided on numbers of athletes treated, typical patterns of physiotherapy intervention, diurnal patterns, areas of highest intensity within the clinic, as well as patterns of injury or illness that could be considered for working toward minimizing incidence in future. Providing

Team XXX Performance Review—objectives and critical incident reflection for CPD

Before leaving for XXX, please think about what you might want to get out of the experience from a personal and professional development perspective. In the box below, list around 4–5 key objectives that you would like to achieve.

Section A: Self Review Form (to be completed by the Appraisee)
Name of Appraisee:
Job Title:
Name of Appraiser:

Please consider key objectives that you expect to achieve within your area of work during the Olympic Games in xxx. Consider how you will measure your success and any CPD activities that may be required to facilitate these objectives.

Part 2 Post-games– Outline areas of your work that you feel have made a positive contribution to your workplace, athlete support and achieving your own objectives. Please consider any factors that may have contributed to this success.

Figure 6.4 Typical template form for objective planning and reflection

Team XXX Performance Review—objectives and critical incident reflection for CPD

Part 3 –Outline areas of your work that you feel could be improved. Please consider any factors that may have impacted on your ability to perform your role to its maximum potential. Is there anything you would have done differently?

Part 4 – What have you learned from the experience to take into your future practice? Can you identify further development objectives to take from this experience?

Figure 6.4 *(Continued)*

- **Calm under pressure**—How well do you feel you dealt with the pressures of working in a games environment? Did you make correct decisions under pressure? Do you think your colleagues thought you appeared calm? Do you think the athletes thought you appeared calm?
- **Awareness of skill level and team mechanics**—Were you able to recognize when you needed to ask for help? Did you use the skills of other members of the team in your management of athletes? Did you feel you were able to adapt your working style depending on who you were working with? Did you feel other team members were comfortable working with you? Were you aware of the different roles and pressures of other team members in wider NOC/sport-specific areas?
- **Focus on performance target**—Were you able to remain focussed on the job in hand i.e., providing a high-quality clinical service? Did you let distractions of being at a games or personal issues get in the way?
- **Personal organization and time keeping**—How well do you think you were able to manage your work and rest times? Were you late for clinic or venue support cover? Were you able to make good use of any available rest time?
- **Ability to perform by adapting to different sporting environments**—How well do you think you were able to change your working style depending on the sport you were working with? Do you think you were aware of/sensitive to different responses to your and adapted your approach appropriately?
- **Clinical knowledge and experience**—Do you feel you had sufficient skills in all areas? Were there things you identified that you would want to work on to improve your breadth/depth of knowledge or skills. Did your previous experiences fully prepare you for this level of sporting environment—what have you learnt on reflection?
- **Interpersonal skills and communication**—How well do you think you integrated with the physio team/medical team/wider team/coaches, and managers, etc. Were you able to communicate assertively but positively with different groups/individuals? Were you sensitive to your position as NOC physio relative to other teams? Was your level of communication appropriate for the environment—e.g., too friendly/not approachable enough—or contributing to discussions letting others speak
- **A team player**—Did you look after your colleagues? Did you do the extra things needed in a games environment that are not typically physiotherapy duties? Did you do them with good grace?!

Figure 6.5 Guidelines for completion of individual performance review

information on work patterns is particularly important for estimating workforce requirements for subsequent Olympic Games, relative to team size and types of sports participating. For instance, identifying where a proportion of work was done, either in the clinic or at the venue, could help explain changes in numbers of contacts, where generally lower numbers of contacts may be identified at the venue compared with the clinic but is something that is an essential area that is more intensive in

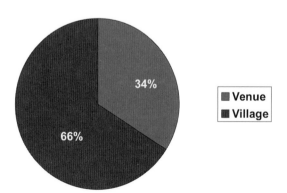

Figure 6.6 Pie chart showing location of treatments

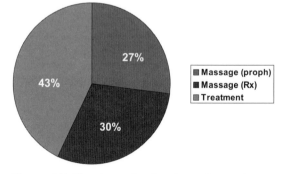

Figure 6.7 Pie chart showing breakdown of massage treatments

staffing numbers (Figure 6.6). Equally a breakdown of treatment approach is likely to show a high proportion of soft tissue work. However, if this work is linked to a concurrent physiotherapeutic treatment as well as for performance, then it could provide useful evidence for the skill mix of the staff required (Figure 6.7).

Suggested reading

Bulley, C., Donaghy, M., Coppoolse, R. *et al.* (2011) *Sports Physiotherapy Competencies*. http://www.ifsp-world.org/public/pdf/Competencies.pdf [accessed March 31, 2011].

Chapter 7
The importance of communication: understanding the importance of the event to the athlete, coach, and others

Bill Moreau[1] and Peter Toohey[2]

[1] United States Olympic Committee, Colorado Springs, CO, USA
[2] United States Olympic Committee, Lake Placid, NY, USA

Introduction

Communication may be defined as:

> ... the activity of conveying meaningful information. Communication requires a sender, a message, and an intended recipient, although the receiver need not be present or aware of the sender's intent to communicate at the time of communication; thus communication can occur across vast distances in time and space. Communication requires that the communicating parties share an area of communicative commonality. The communication process is complete once the receiver has understood the sender (Wikipedia 2011).

Each of us interacts in thousands of communications each day. The steadily increasing volume of communication may lead us to jump to the conclusion that the communication process must be an easy task implemented through a seamless process. Unidirectional messaging is indeed easy; however, effective communication is more often a much more complex process that requires planning, skills, and an overlying strategy. The process of communicating or receiving communications regarding what appears to be an extremely straightforward idea may result in frustration, misunderstanding, and dysfunction. In sports medicine, dysfunctional communication may result in important problems for any or all parties involved in the communication process. Effective communication may represent one of the most complex and valuable tasks that comprises the field of sports medicine. The goal of this chapter is to provide some overlying best practices and clinical pearls to help the clinician structure and effectively send and receive *meaningful information* or communications in sports medicine.

Developing a sports medicine communication strategy

Developing a sports medicine communication strategy involves several important considerations that should be addressed in advance of the need for implementation of that strategy. Sports medicine communication involves many people who represent internal and external partners to the athlete. Each partner's role or involvement with the athlete is not always clear.

Sports Therapy Services, First Edition. Edited by James E. Zachazewski and David J. Magee.
© 2012 International Olympic Committee. Published 2012 by John Wiley & Sons, Ltd.

Internal partners are primarily health care providers who are directly providing care to the athlete. Examples of internal providers would include but is not limited to the athlete's primary care physician, physiotherapist, chiropractor, orthopedic surgeon, or sport's psychologist. The athlete's internal partners should share information regarding the individual athletes' health status to develop a team approach to the athlete's care. An exception would be when the athlete specifically identifies confidential information that he or she does not want to be communicated to others.

External partners are composed of those groups of individuals who have a vested interest in the athlete's health status but are not directly involved in the delivery of health care services. These groups of people or organizations will present different levels of complexity in regard to communication of the athlete's health status. More often than not, the health care team will need to consult with the athlete before discussing health information with external partners. This permission is required due to the confidential nature of much of this information.

Some groups of individuals can be considered both an internal and external partner. Good examples would include the athlete's coach and National Governing Body (NGB). As individuals, they may not have direct access to the athlete's health care status, but most likely these two groups will be in-

volved in large press conferences and internal sporting decisions regarding team selection and strategy around athlete availability for competitions.

Figure 7.1 depicts the internal and external partners involved in athlete communication issues. The athlete is the center of the hub of communication in regard to clinical care or event preparations. Internal communications are defined as those communications that occur within the "protected confines of the sports medicine organizational structure." The athlete's family, coaches, and "sports organizations" may or may not be included in protected communications. The inclusion or exclusion would be based on the rules that are in place. Examples of rules in sports include sports organization communications such as boxing commissions, NGBs, and athletic associations that have recognized doctrine in place for the athlete regarding the communication of sports medicine-related issues. The IOC has established anti-doping rules, expecting that, in the spirit of sport, these rules will contribute to the fight against doping in the Olympic movement. The rules are complemented by other IOC documents and international standards addressed throughout the rules.

Additional variables need to be weighed when considering these partners access to information about the athlete's medical status, especially at a critical time such as the Olympic Games. Some considerations include the age of the athlete, sporting

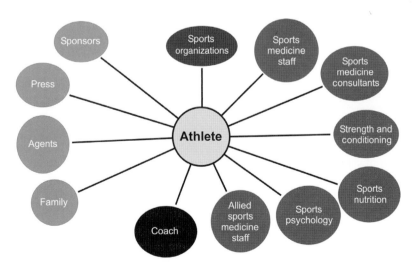

Figure 7.1 Internal and external communication partners in sports medicine

rules, and the athlete's personal wishes. Recognize that all of these partners have their own internal interests in gaining information. It is of utmost importance to identify the legal permissions, athlete's wishes, timing, and the specific individual who will communicate information and the depth of information to be revealed in advance of the disclosure of any health care information.

There are three key components that all health care providers need to recognize regarding communications with athletes who present for care (Brown and Bylund 2008):

1 Effective communication skills in athlete and coach interactions are linked to important athlete outcomes.

2 One should not assume that communication skills are always optimal; therefore, athlete care outcomes can be improved.

3 Communication skills can be taught and learned.

The concept that "You can never over communicate" is often heard. In this day of rapid communication with hundreds of daily e-mails, blogs, text messages, and instant messaging passing back and forth, this old adage may not still hold true. How many of you actually avoid sifting through the e-mails from colleagues who are over communicators? Today the best adage may be you need to succinctly communicate until the message is conveyed. The volume of communication does not necessarily equate with effectiveness in communication.

The skills and abilities to efficiently decipher salient incoming information and subsequently craft a succinct, linear response message are critical and is a learned skill. This type of message includes enough information to allow your message to be understood and not serve as a distraction or confuse the issue the communication is about. If the sender does not construct his or her message effectively, the receiver of a message may complain that the message was confusing or incomplete while the sender of the message may feel frustrated or disappointed that the receiver could not correctly interpret the message. Interactive communication requires at least two people to be involved in the communication with a solution-oriented approach.

The volume of communication flow from multiple sources regarding an athletes' health care

Table 7.1 Examples of types of communication pipelines in sports medicine

Oral communication	E-mail
Fax	Letters
Clinical entries	Press
Texting	Instant messaging
Telephone conversations	Staff meetings
Seminars	Consultant reports
Body language	Research
Manuscripts	Position papers
Rules and regulations	Conferences

status can be significant, sometimes resulting in what might be considered an overflow (Table 7.1). If not controlled, filtered, and prioritized, the volume of communication may present substantial obstacles for the sports medicine team. In order to best manage the information, each person or organization should develop a strategic approach to information management. There are many strategies that have been promoted for information management. Some of these common strategies include the following:

Touch It Once: Time management experts recommend the "touch it once" method for effectiveness and efficiency. The idea is that when you receive a message in the form of a letter, e-mail, or voice mail, you complete the task and then you can move on to the next task.

Lists: Some experts recommend that you make and maintain lists of tasks to be completed and then attack the lists based on the priority of the task.

Time: This approach includes planning your day to complete the most important task first thing in the morning before you open the information pipeline.

These approaches may make sense for the executive; however, the implementation of the management strategy in everyday life may become much more difficult for busy sports medicine health care providers who have clinical duties that consume the majority of their day along with the inevitable urgent interruptions. Each individual needs to identify a process that best works for him or her.

The originator and responder of a communication must formulate thought, identify the audience, weigh the priority of the initiative, check for organizational alignment, identify potential conflicts, and then create an effective communication. This process can occur in less than a second through facial expressions, or spoken responses, or require months when the message represents an organizational position or planning for a major athletic event.

Effectively managing information, absorbing messaging and tracking ongoing communications, requires time, attention, and other resources to be successful. In today's world of information overflow, the ability to rapidly filter the information overload in order to identify important information is quickly becoming a cornerstone for defining success.

Collaborative communication

Effective communication requires one to collaborate with the communication partners in both the delivery and reception of information while simultaneously understanding the other partner(s) perspectives. Personal and organizational level communications each have their own unique challenges that require skill sets that change to meet the audience regardless of whether one is the originator or responder to the communication.

Building collaborative communication does not always just happen. Feudtner (2007) has identified the following five tasks for building collaborative communication:

1 Establish common goals to guide collaborative efforts.
2 Exhibit mutual respect and compassion for each other.
3 Develop a sufficiently complete understanding of our differing perspectives.
4 Assure maximum clarity and correctness of what we communicate to each other.
5 Manage intrapersonal and interpersonal processes that affect how we send, receive, and process information.

When one is communicating to multiple parties including organizations, athletes, coaches, other sports medicine staff, the public, or the press, one must be able to quickly customize his or her communication skill sets. The same message may have different meanings to the recipient depending on the audience. Each recipient of the message will interpret the communication based on multiple factors including prior experiences with the writer, age, educational background, culture, native language, preferred methods of communication, and his or her personal perspective.

Another key point is to ensure that multiple divergent messages are not coming out of the same sports medicine department. This issue will be discussed further in Section "Sports Medicine Team Communications" of this chapter.

There are fundamental ways that communication takes place. Today, people are quickly connected through more channels or communication pipelines than ever before. It is common practice to have many forms of routine communication daily that include international partners. The explosion of the communication pipeline is going to only expand from where we are today.

Even a single individual can act as a hub for sports medicine communication because of his or her unique expertise, employment position, or role as an opinion maker. People may form ties for many reasons including specific attributes such as individuals who are interested in a particular field of sports medicine like concussion or the female athlete triad. Reaching out to like-minded individuals in the field of sports medicine that share interests can be a very valuable endeavor.

There are also readily identifiable useful networks of communication in sports medicine that can save time and provide answers to questions. The sports communication network may range from large-scale sports medicine social groups to very tight focused athlete to clinician communications.

It may be useful for the individual sports medicine provider to seek out others with similar interests to best provide the most streamlined access to advance the individual's specific area of interest. The ability to identify new information that is pertinent to the individual's area of interest is a substantial challenge. One of the most effective methods to expand ones sports medicine network is to attend educational conferences and symposiums.

Athlete communications

The most important customer of the sports medicine communication process is the athlete. The athlete may be the individual the communication is directed to, received from, or they may be the beneficiaries of the communications between other parties. Clinicians should never underestimate the importance of the two-way communication street of effective communication.

There are many components to earning and keeping an athlete's trust. One way is to improve the communication between sports medicine staff and the athlete. Consistent and positive behavior is also a fundamental component of developing trust. Another way is to empathize with the athlete. It is alright to respond to the athlete's emotion. The linkage between the health care provider and the athlete can be encouraged by allowing the athlete to express his or her feelings and by providing hope and reassurance.

According to Diermeier (2011), many factors influence trust. Some are based on rational, cognitive factors and some are based on nonrational emotional factors. Consider the following four factors to obtain or restore the trust of an athlete: clinical expertise, commitment, informed consent, and transparency. In sports medicine, it makes sense that clinicians will find their greatest comfort zone within the area of clinical expertise in convincing the athlete of his or her competency. Commitment in communicating that the problem will be addressed and there is a clear process in place that will address the issue. This communication is best delivered by the individual in charge. Empathy should be an area of focused attention. The clinician should be perceived with a warm and empathetic attitude. One should also not underestimate the importance of transparency in telling the athlete what one knows, what one does not know, and when one will follow up with them (Figure 7.2).

Athletes expect and deserve clinical expertise in the management of their illness or injury. Clinical competency is a key to not only clinical outcomes but also to creating a trusting environment for the athlete. Just like health care in the public sector, if

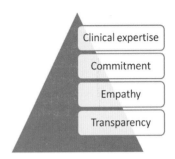

Figure 7.2 The trust pyramid (Adapted from Diermeier (2011))

the patient does not trust the health care provider's assessment and care plan, the relationship is already on shaky ground.

It is not just the elite professional or Olympic level athlete who is fully committed to their sport. Athletes from many walks of life see sport as a large component of their identity. High-level athletes expect the same level of commitment to sport from the sports medicine staff as they give as participants. The quickest way to demonstrate commitment is to be there when one says one will be there. Covering or visiting practices may not seem that enticing, but it demonstrates you, as an individual, are also in it to help the athlete win! An athlete should be able to expect sincerity from all members of the sports medicine team. Many a relationship has been damaged by one quick slip. Sincerity is best conveyed through one's oral communications and body language. It is hard to sell that an individual is sincerely interested in the athlete when that individual is accessing their e-mail and sending instant messages while the athlete is speaking to them. Make sure if you are simultaneously researching what the athlete is talking to you about that you make the athlete aware of what you are doing.

Informed consent is an excellent opportunity to provide information and include the athlete in the care pathway for his or her illness or injury. Sports medicine providers should not expect protection from informed consent doctrine because they are in a somewhat unique care setting. Using a paternal versus patient-centered approach when working with elite athletes is most likely an ill-advised

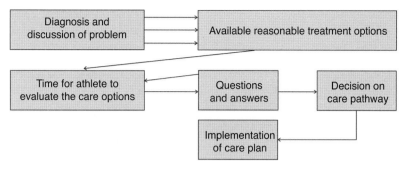

Figure 7.3 Basic model of communicating informed consent

approach to care. The basic model of informed consent is depicted in Figure 7.3.

Any diagnosis should be accurate and openly disclosed to the athlete along with the possible action plans to treat the condition. The athlete should be allowed to consider the information and then be allowed to ask additional questions so he or she can best select the care pathway that makes the most sense to him or her. In obvious emergent situations, this processing occurs much more quickly, or not at all, if the athlete's life may be in jeopardy. In Olympic and other elite level sports, the timelines to participate in the next qualifying event are important and the athlete's concern over these types of issues should not be negated.

Open and transparent communication is a must in sports medicine. Transparent communication regarding decision making that incorporates the athlete allows for the mutual accountability of the clinician and the athlete to be held accountable to each other. Transparency in communication activities involves clearly describing the athlete's problems and the subsequent care plan for the patient. The basics include the identification of the diagnosis, possible clinical pathways, informed consent, and expected resultant goals of care that include a timeline.

Another key to effective communication is to understand the preferred form of communications the athletes use. Believe it or not, e-mail was once considered advanced communication! Today some athletes do not even check their e-mail and they will only respond to instant messaging. Make sure that you can lawfully disclose information by electronic media before doing so. The media the athletes use

may determine if you are able to get the meaningful communication loop closed.

Working with athletes who are minors represents additional challenges in the communication process. At high-level sporting activities, it is not uncommon for the athlete to not have a parent with them when they present for care. The laws of the country, region, or state will dictate the specific nuances regarding the care you can provide to minors. Health care providers need to know these laws before they are engaged in care. Young individuals are not always accurate when they relay their health care information to a provider on the physical form. Whenever possible, have a parent or guardian of the athlete confirm that the history is correct.

Young athlete patients may want to know information from their health care provider team, but they may lack the self-confidence to ask a direct question that addresses the issue. Watch for body language or indirect questions to help identify the possible request for additional information as you communicate. The young patient may say "I really don't know much about what you are talking about." This type of statement is an indication that the patient is asking to learn more.

Steps for the successful patient communication process

1 Evaluate the Environment. Ensure that you are in a secure listening area when you are verbally communicating important or sensitive information to the athlete. Recognize that you may receive different answers to your questions dependent upon who is in the area when you are talking to the athlete or provide your report of findings. An athlete surrounded by his or her teammates or coach may provide a much different answer to your questions than an athlete who is in a secure conversation area. When possible move your discussions to a quiet controlled area.

2 Confirm You Are Connected. Face the athlete, make and hold eye contact with the athlete when conversing. Observe the athlete for body language, such as an affirmative nodding of the head, to confirm you are connecting with your message. Reinforce to the athlete that he or she is involved and that identifying the clinical pathway of care is a joint decision-making process. Recognize that there is a wide variability in individuals and there are many markers of "closing the loop" in the communication process.

3 Speak in Understandable Terminology. Use terms the athlete knows and can understand. Avoid using technical anatomical and medical terminology unless it is a necessary part of the conversation. The use of drawings and diagrams that the athlete can review with you and then take with him or her is a useful tool to improve communication.

4 Order of Delivering the Message. Communicate the most important aspect of the message first and reinforce this message at the end of the conversation.

    a Provide and explain the diagnosis.

    b Identify the exam and history findings that support your diagnosis (e.g., physical examination findings, imaging reports, mechanism of injury).

    c List the care options, while identifying each options and their advantages and disadvantages, then identify the recommended care option.

    d Identify and explain which option you think is the best pathway to follow. Understand the athlete may choose not to follow this path.

    e Include the risks, benefits, and estimated return to play timeline for the care pathway.

    f Communicate the necessary steps or markers to be met for the return to play process.

    g Attempt to define the return to play timeline.

5 Encourage the Athlete to Interrupt You If He or She Has Any Questions. Ask on more than one occasion if the athlete has questions. If there are many questions, you may not be presenting the case in a linear or logical fashion or you may be communicating at a level above the individual's level of understanding. Remember, the athlete will be the one who determines if you are clearly communicating.

6 Confirm the Communication Loop Is Completed. Ask the athlete to tell you in his or her own words what he or she thinks you have just communicated to him or her. Allow the athlete to completely formulate and finish his or her thoughts before correcting misinformation. Summarize the discussion by identifying the key components of the history, exam, diagnosis, selected care plan, any associated risks, and next steps.

7 Provide Clearly Written Instructions. The use of forms to communicate and summarize the athlete's encounter is an essential task. The athlete should not be expected to articulate to others a complex injury discussion that involves multiple variables. Ensure that you have received permission from the athlete as to whom you may and may not communicate with regarding to his or her injury or illness. After considering the classifications of his or her sport, be sure to identify the return to play process and level of activity that the athlete may participate in.

Coach communications

The ability to clearly communicate and collaborate with your coaching staff is an essential skill for health care providers in sports medicine. The recognition of the coaches' preferred method of communication is a good first step. Understand coaches' need to have current and timely communications from the sports medicine staff in order to make decisions based on the health status of the athlete(s) they supervise. This may not be as simple a process as it first appears.

Games communications

Communication between the National Olympic Committee (NOC) and Local Organizing

Committee (LOC) is the foundation to a successful international games competition. The symbiotic relationship between the two parties takes substantial time to develop and grow. At the highest level of communication, the IOC is in constant communication with the LOC to monitor the progress of developing the games support. Time wise, the areas of communication regarding sports medicine are included from when the bid for an Olympic Games is received to the closing ceremonies. Developing and then communicating a well-constructed sports medicine plan provides for a platform of confidence to an NOC in developing their IOC relationship. Establishing a rapport is critical and identifying a communication style to suit both parties is a necessary first step. Several considerations must be taken into account, such as geographical, cultural, environmental, and logistical factors, all of which will expand the relationship as the timeline gets closer to the opening ceremonies. It is through communicating a structured timeline that is developed by the IOC and the LOC, which will initially solidify the expectations of both parties and wiliness to collaborate toward a common goal.

Games communication strategy

When an international games bid is granted by the IOC to a LOC, a direct report is established. In turn, the LOC assigns a delegate to each NOC to assure a personal contact. Each NOC determines the best communication structure to accommodate their nation. Communication between the LOC and NOC will vary from face-to-face meetings at venue site visits to telephone and electronic mail. An onsite visit of the village or test event at a venue scheduled prior to the actual international games competition presents all parties with an excellent opportunity for the NOC to discuss with the LOC any adjustment that can result in successful games. At this point of preparedness, having specific job descriptions for key rolls within the NOC is suggested. For example, the LOC will name a chief medical officer (CMO) and each NOC will name a CMO. Interacting and communicating at specific venue sites during "test" competitions leading up

to the Olympic Games can allow CMOs and staff at all levels to make any final adjustments needed in emergency protocol.

The host CMO will be the hub of communication regarding medical issues. Each individual country will have their CMO who will look to the host country CMO for guidance regarding all aspects of setting up the medical services for the games. Also, it allows LOC and NOC medical staff to partner in developing further relationships. Communication at every level from the Chef de Mission to individual service providers is necessary when developing an overall sports medicine communication strategy.

Primary communication

The IOC sets a standard and supervises the progress of the LOC when hosting an international games event. The LOC has flexibility in logistics, but the standards, such as the polyclinic locations in each International village, nutritional considerations accommodated by the village staff, doping procedures and process, and local resources for credentialed versus noncredentialed personnel, are the primary communication contacts that need to be established. Other contact considerations to improve communication at the games are illustrated in Table 7.2.

The LOC will publish contact personnel information and job responsibilities that you should be aware of. Critical individuals are as follows:
- **Chef de Mission:** NOC representative to the LOC and IOC at an international games. All communication will be directed from the LOC/IOC to

Table 7.2 Critical communication considerations

• National embassy	• Venue directors
• Repatriation (the process of returning the individual back to their place of citizenship if they die or if they are severely injured)	• Local hospitals
	• Insurance protection
	• Security contact
	• Air and ground transportation
• Customs process (for import and export shipping)	

NOC through daily meetings from opening to closing ceremonies. For example, if a doping violation is found during competition, the first person to be notified will be the Chef de Mission of each NOC.

- **Chief Medical Officer:** The LOC will appoint a CMO. Their primary responsibility is to oversee and establish medical services during the international games. The CMO will be the primary medical contact between LOC–CMO and the NOC–CMO.
- **Chief Doping Officer (CDO):** The LOC will collaborate with the World Anti-Doping Agency (WADA) to assure proper procedures and process is flawless during competition.
- **Venue Director(s):** LOC venue directors will work with CMO and CDO in order to accommodate services including emergency action plan. The LOC polyclinic directors will work with the CMOs to streamline medical services including emergency and transportation. Multiple LOC personnel will assist in the NOC's success at an international games event.

Secondary communication

Internal communication is a necessity for an NOC to present their culture to the world through sporting competition. Creating a team within an NOC, which has direct knowledge of the success of their sports, will result in greater understanding of the needs in a foreign environment. Having the NOC team meet the direct contacts at the LOC will strengthen the information between your internal team. The NOC team structure should emulate the LOCs and any other considerations should be made in the interest of improving performance of the NOC's athletes. Position of consideration: Chef de Mission, Assistant Chef de Mission, Chief Medical Officer, Medical Director, Village Director, Chief Council, Chief of Security, High Performance Directors, and third-party support systems.

The local chief medical officer (CMO/LOC) is tasked to maintain international relationships, as well as directing each individual sports medicine staff. The CMO/LOC must communicate with each individual sport and country to identify the medical services and personnel necessary for each sport to perform successfully. The personnel component

is important—for example, a bobsled athlete is going to have different needs than a figure skater.

Constant communications between the CMO and each sports-specific medical staff is critical due to the limited number of credentials available during the international games. Situation will arise where there will not be enough credentials to support every team. The CMO will need to identify any gaps in services and accommodate with more diverse medical staff. For example, if alpine skiing was given two credentials for medical, but Nordic combine does not have any credentials for medical, it would be wise to have the two medical staff with alpine assist with Nordic combine as well. The CMO needs to use multiple communication resources to be effective leading up to the games and through closing ceremonies.

Communication strategy is going to be an evolving project from the start to the finish of an international event. Collaboration between LOC and NOC will assure resources are efficiently used, teamwork between NOC personnel will establish a structure for athletes and coaches to rely upon, and the harmony of the Olympic movement will inspire people of the world.

Sports medicine team communications

The sports medicine team needs to have a plan in place for a communication strategy. Substantial frustration by all parties is a sure consequence of not developing a sports medicine communication strategy. When the members of the sports medicine team must have respect for each other, communication pipelines (see Table 7.1) will naturally occur to the athlete's benefit. The steps to develop a communication plan in the sports medicine department will need to be initiated by the director of the sports medicine clinic with substantial input from the whole sports medicine team. A clinic director who fails to incorporate open discussion from the entire sports medicine team will likely lose a prime opportunity to create alignment of the sports medicine team.

The overall communication strategy regardless if it is for implementation at the clinic, CMO, head

Table 7.3 Communication check list

When does the clinic director or individual in charge of an athlete expect to be informed of an athlete's injury?	• Any referral to an urgent care center? • When the athlete does not improve within a specified period of time? • If there is a diagnosis of a head or spinal injury? • When there is syncope or chest pain during or after an exercise bout? • If there is a personal issue between the athlete and staff?
How does the clinic director prefer to receive urgent and nonurgent communications?	• By cell phone 24/7? • Instant messaging or e-mail? • Fax?
Who may disclose an athlete's diagnosis and status relative to continued participation?	• Any member of the sports medicine staff? • Only team physician/CMO? • Only coach of team?
Who may make return to play decisions?	• Any member of the sports medicine staff? • Only team physician/CMO? • Only coach of team?
Who is contacted in an emergent situation when the clinic director is out of communication?	• Is there a preestablished chain of command?
Who may communicate and interpret to the athlete special test findings such as diagnostic imaging, laboratory results, and pulmonary function testing?	• Any member of the sports medicine staff? • Only team physician/CMO?

physician, coach, or all the way up to the Chef de Mission can be assessed using the check list illustrated in Table 7.3.

Public relations strategy

It is important to remember you may lose the privilege of representing your independent thoughts through public communications when you are a member of a sports medicine organization within the auspices of a larger organization such as the country's NOC, an Olympic team, a professional team, or college team. Depending on the topic addressed and the role you hold within an organization, the organization may place restrictions on what and how you communicate on a specific topic. It is easy to understand how your personal communications and positions could, and most likely will, be extrapolated to represent the position of the organization that employs or retains you. A good rule of thumb is to run through your organization's press relations and legal department outside communications regarding areas of policy or potential controversy in advance.

This is particularly true in a setting such as a news conference or one-on-one interview where you are officially representing your organization (Figure 7.4). That is not to say that you should misinform anyone, especially a member of the media. However, there are instances where the full details of an athlete's injury may impact the preparation of the larger team and it is inappropriate to divulge your full medical diagnosis or the treatment being given.

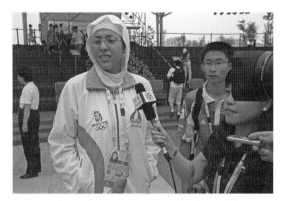

Figure 7.4 Press interview at Beijing Games (Photo courtesy of the International Olympic Committee)

Even more important to consider when dealing with the media is that each question asked is an opportunity for you to deliver the message of your choosing. You can and should appropriately answer the journalist's question, but you should also take that opportunity to expand your comments. For instance, if asked whether or not an athlete is fit for competition. You may be tempted to simply say, "Yes." However, it is also an opportunity for speaking to the athlete's preparation and training. You are part of a bigger organization and the comments from a medical standpoint need to stand by themselves. But any time you have the opportunity to positively affect the brand of your organization, you should take it. In an ever-changing media landscape, an athlete, team, or organization's brand is impacted by the comments of every person associated with said athlete, team, or organization, and the sponsorships, donations, and the overall reputation of the organization depend on positive, exhibited traits.

Another thing to consider is that *you are never off the record*. Not only that, but in an era of ubiquitous mobile phone cameras and video recording devices, nearly everything you do and say in a games environment may appear in public, whether it is a news organization's Web site or simply a post on someone's favorite social media forum. Citizen journalism is now the norm and you should consider yourself on the record at all times.

Crisis communication skills

Crisis communication is critically important to the success of your organization in a   difficult time. The most important factors to successful crisis communication are to be prepared, accurate and available.

You cannot plan for every scenario, but you can plan the process you will use in a crisis. Once you gather the first set of facts available (and those facts will no doubt change), you need a plan in place for who in your organizational chain of command should be notified and in what order. You should continue to gather facts and constantly communicate any updates to the appropriate people.

Your public relations staff will take the lead in communicating the relevant facts to the media and beyond, but they must have the most relevant facts available to ensure that they remain a trusted source of information. It is near impossible to regain the trust of the media or the general public once it is gone, so timely, fact-based communication is key.

References

Brown, R.F. & Bylund, C.L. (2008) Communication skills training: describing a new conceptual model. *Academic Medicine*, 83(1), 37–44.

Diermeier, D. (2011) *Reputation Rules: Strategies for Building Your Company's Most Valuable Asset*. McGraw Hill, New York.

Feudtner, C. (2007) Collaborative communication in pediatric palliative care: a foundation for problem-solving and decision-making. *Pediatric Clinics of North America*, 54(5), 583–ix.

Wikipedia: The Free Encyclopedia, http://en.wikipedia.org/wiki/Communication. Accessed September 13, 2011.

Chapter 8

Considerations for working with professional athletes versus nonprofessional amateur athletes during Olympic events

Sergio T. Fonseca[1], Juliana Melo Ocarino[1], Thales Rezende Souza[1], Anderson Aurélio da Silva[1], José Roberto Prado Jr[2], Natália Franco Netto Bittencourt[1], and Luciana De Michelis Mendonça[1]

[1]Universidade Federal De Minas Gerais, Belo Horizonte, MG, Brazil
[2]Centro Universitário Augusto Motta, RJ, Brazil

Introduction

The Olympic Games represent a great challenge for athletes who usually prepare themselves for a long time and in a very intense way. The routine of training and the great demand during Olympic events induce an increased risk of musculoskeletal injury (Junge *et al.* 2008; Badekas *et al.* 2009). During the Athens Olympic Games in 2004, for example, the musculoskeletal injuries included overuse injuries (e.g., general tendinopathies, patellofemoral dysfunction) and acute injuries (e.g., ligament sprain and muscle strain, fractures), and most of these injuries affected the lower extremities (Badekas *et al.* 2009; Athanasopoulos *et al.* 2007). The specific diagnosis of sprain/strain was the most common reason for visiting medical care at the Olympic Games in 1996 (Wetterhall *et al.* 1998) and in 2008 (Junge *et al.* 2009). In addition, in Beijing in 2008, there was an incidence of 96.1 injuries per 1000 registered athletes. The majority of these injuries (72.5%) occurred during competition and half of them prevented athlete participation in training or competition (Junge *et al.* 2009). This relative high incidence of injuries during the Olympic Games poses a great

demand on the sport therapist. Thus, the occurrence of injuries and the process of rehabilitation of the injured athlete have been an important subject for international sports federations and for the International Olympic Committee (IOC), which combine efforts to establish standardized surveillance of sports injuries not only to provide epidemiological information but also to direct efforts to injury prevention (Junge *et al.* 2009).

Injury prevention and rehabilitation programs designed for Olympic athletes are essential for their proper performance. However, due to the fact that athletes competing at the Olympic Games sometimes do not have similar levels of care and attention by the medical team and that the care they receive varies in terms of training infrastructure available to them, the role of the sports therapist in the development of these programs is quite dependent upon the context of the athlete's practice. Usually, professional athletes, who are able to participate in the Olympics, are highly paid to compete and have at their disposal the best medical/health care infrastructure possible in terms of equipment and highly skilled and knowledgeable personnel. Although a truely amateur athlete very often does not have a regular source of income and does not have access to the medical/health care infrastructure available to the professional. However, some successful amateur athletes have enough financial support to access necessary services for training and injury management in order to make and participate in Olympic events. These Olympic-level amateur athletes may have a professional infrastructure around them. Thus, in addition to the challenge of attending the Olympic athlete, sports therapist must be prepared to deal with important differences in terms of the logistical working conditions and expectations of each group of athletes.

In order to address the role of the sports therapist in dealing with athletes with different profiles, this chapter is organized into two main sections. The first section will discuss the challenge of the sports therapist when working with athletes, especially in terms of proper clinical reasoning for injury prevention and rehabilitation. In addition, this section will present the expectations and context of paid professional athletes and nonpaid amateur athletes. The second section will discuss the impact and role of private sports therapists who care for professional athletes compared with sports therapists who are part of official sports medicine team provided by the country for the competition.

Working with athletes

To work with athletes, the sports therapist should understand the athlete's context and the processes involved in injury production. Musculoskeletal injuries occur when the amount of energy applied to a particular tissue exceeds a critical limit. Despite this simple concept, the occurrence of injuries has a multifactorial nature with contribution and complex interactions of many biomechanical factors. The capability of the musculoskeletal system of the athlete to deal with different stress demands arising during sporting activity determines whether or not a given pathological condition occurs. Thus, the sports therapist must be able to understand the complex nature of the injury in order to provide the best care possible to the Olympic athlete.

In this section, a brief theoretical consideration that guides the therapist's clinical reasoning required to assist the athlete and a discussion about the sport context in which the therapist acts are presented.

Clinical reasoning for injury prevention and rehabilitation of athletes

During training or competition, the whole body (i.e., the kinetic chain) of the athlete is subjected to internal (i.e., muscle, inertial, and joint intersegmental forces) and external forces (i.e., ground reaction and impact forces) that have to be dissipated or transferred appropriately among body segments and tissues, so as to guarantee movement efficiency and structural integrity (Fonseca et al. 2007). As the musculoskeletal system works as a kinetic chain, joints transmit forces among segments. This force transmission mechanism is possible due to the mechanical linkages between bones and seems to depend on the anatomic and functional continuity among the connective tissue of fascia, muscles, ligaments, and tendons (for more detail on force transmission in the kinetic chain, read Vleeming et al. 1995; Zajac et al. 2002; Huijing and Jaspers 2005; Myers 2009). The appropriate mechanical energy flow generated by force transmission redistributes energy within the body and between the body and the environment. Inadequate energy distribution (e.g., energy concentration on a tissue/joint or poor energy dissipation) throughout the kinetic chain is among the main factors responsible for injury production (Fonseca et al. 2007).

The capability of the musculoskeletal system to generate, transfer, and dissipate mechanical energy constitutes the individual's dynamic resources (Fonseca et al. 2004). The amount of energy the tissue can absorb is related to its susceptibility to injury (Butler et al. 2003). The greater the tissue capacity of energy absorption (i.e., area under the stress–strain curve), the lower the susceptibility to injury (Akeson et al. 1984). Properties such as muscle endurance, tissue stiffness, muscle length, and eccentric force determine the capability of the biological tissue to absorb energy (Butler et al. 2003; Garrett et al. 1987). In addition, appropriate muscle and joint stiffness are properties required to allow efficient energy transfer among segments of the kinetic chain necessary to generate appropriate movement patterns (Fonseca *et al.* 2007). In this context, not only the capability of the muscles to generate force, as traditionally considered, but also muscles' (and other tissues) capability to dissipate and transfer energy among body segments should be the main concern of the sports therapist during the athletes' rehabilitation and injury prevention processes.

During sports activities, the musculoskeletal system of the athlete is subjected to demands arising from specificities of the sport activity and of the body structure. In this context, working with athletes involves, initially, a specific knowledge of the athlete's activity-related demands, since movement patterns involved in sport activity can impose excessive stresses on the musculoskeletal system of the athlete. The magnitude of these stresses depends on characteristics such as level of competition and training, type of sport, equipment use, activity duration, and movement speed. For this reason, the type and frequency of injuries are different among sports. At the Athens Olympic Games, severe injuries such as ligament sprains or bone fractures were more frequent in soccer, basketball, volleyball, and handball compared with other sports (Badekas *et al.* 2009).

In addition to the activity-related demand, the musculoskeletal systems of the athletes are subjected to specific stress demands related to their body structure (Fonseca *et al.* 2007). Anatomic characteristics such as altered biomechanical alignment can increase the stress demand in particular biological tissues or specific joints of the kinetic chain. For example, rearfoot and forefoot varus alignment may cause compensatory and excessive movements at particular joints (e.g., excessive femur internal rotation) during activities performed with the foot fixed on the ground, which may lead to increased stress on biological tissues (Michaud 1993). Therefore, the sports therapist must know not only the sport in which the athlete is involved but also the structural characteristics and potentials of the athlete's musculoskeletal system.

Since the relationship between the individual capability and the demand applied on the muscu-loskeletal system determines whether or not a given pathological condition occurs (see Fonseca *et al.* 2010 for soccer examples), prevention and rehabilitation programs established by the sports therapist should involve strategies to optimize the athlete's capabilities and/or to minimize the demand on the biological tissues. In this context, the sports therapists' clinical reasoning should be focused on four main topics:

1 The complex musculoskeletal system's anatomical and biomechanical properties and the role of these properties in the generation, dissipation, and transfer of mechanical energy.

2 The demands on the musculoskeletal system arising from the specific sport activity and from the body structure.

3 How the musculoskeletal system generates and adapts to different interactions among body segments. Specifically, the biomechanical and functional relationships among anatomically adjacent and remote body parts.

4 The biomechanics of the whole kinetic chain and how it is related to performance and injury occurrence.

Considering the complex nature of the injury process, in which extensive knowledge of the sport and athlete is required, the sports therapist is faced with a great challenge when providing care for an Olympic team. While in an ideal world, the care provided to professionals and amateurs would be identical, the reality is that paid professional athletes and nonpaid amateur athletes may receive different care from the sports medicine team and have different expectations in terms of the care provided based on their ability to access and pay for care.

The sport context: professionals versus amateurs

Sports therapists must consider the context in which paid professional and amateur athletes act (Olympic level or not), when planning rehabilitation and/or prevention programs (Goforth *et al.* 2007). Aspects such as personal expectations and external control by sponsors or employers impose different demands on professional and amateur athletes. The context of practice for Olympic athletes involves a systematized training program and a wide support from the health care team (Nosfinger 2007) and from coaches in the training settings (Goforth et al. 2007). In addition, these athletes have at their disposal better infrastructure in terms of equipment and training environment. Therefore, the professional or amateur athletes who participate in Olympic Games often undergo greater pressure for results and performance improvement (Pensgaard & Ursin 1998).

The context of the amateur and professional athletes may be quite different or very similar, depending on several factors. An example of a distinction between amateur and professional athletes is that amateur athletes are, in general, under less pressure for results than the professional ones, since they often have a less structured training environment and less financial support. Amateur athletes must dedicate time simultaneously to their occupation/job and to their sport of choice. In addition, coaches and the medical team may not work full time with the amateur athlete and, frequently, are not present during training sections. For this reason, the training routine depends on the level of commitment of the amateur athletes to follow the recommendations of the professionals who may assist them. Differently, in special cases, amateur athletes have financial support provided by sponsors, which allows them to obtain more organized structure of training and access to health care professionals, similarly to professional athletes. These "special" amateur athletes have better conditions to achieve higher performance levels, which in turn may allow them to succeed and be able to participate in Olympic events. Thus, while the attention to the amateur athlete may be influenced by the limitation of the available infrastructure and work organization, the sports therapist attending professionals or better structured amateur athletes has to deal with interests arising not only from other members of the health care team (Pensgaard & Ursin 1998) but mainly from sponsors and team directors (Thelwell et al. 2008).

Given the context-dependent distinctions and similarities of working with professional and amateur athletes, an overview of the specific context of the sports therapist who work with these athletes and the respective athletes' expectations are presented.

Working with professional athletes

The organizational structure in which an athlete is inserted may vary among different sports and among teams from the same sport (Goforth et al. 2007). This may also differ depending on the level of funding and sophistication of the sport or league (e.g., professional baseball compared with professional soccer or lacrosse in the United States). In general, the sports therapist is a member of the official sports medicine team and can provide care in four areas: (1) emergency care, since the sports medicine professional is present at the majority of training sessions and trips; (2) rehabilitation; (3) functional return; and (4) injury prevention during the preseason and throughout the championships (Silva et al. 2011). Furthermore, the sports therapist is in charge of communicating with the other members of the medical team about the physical condition of the player, focusing on meeting the athlete's real capability to the expectations, pressures, and demands imposed by the team and the club.

Considering the multifactorial nature of injuries, the sports therapist must work within a multidisciplinary context (Elphinston & Hardman 2006; Burke 1995). The organizational structure involved in attention to the professional athlete allows sports therapist access and the ability to work closely with other professionals (e.g., nutritionists, psychologists, and sports medicine teams). This teamwork can promote treatment and prevention programs more efficiently than may be possible for an amateur athlete. In addition to work with other professionals of the health care team, the sports therapist's preventive actions depend on the competition calendar and on the involvement of the team staff, since one of the challenges is to insert preventive work into a routine of several training sessions, matches, and trips. For this reason, the sports therapist should make it clear to coaches and trainers that these interventions are aimed at adjusting the capacity of the athlete's musculoskeletal system to meet the demands imposed by his or her specific sport, with the major purpose of improving performance and decreasing susceptibility to injury. Specific discussions about the role of the sports therapist during pre-event, event, and post-event phases are presented in Chapter 3.

The organizational/logistics structure available to professional athletes allows them to fully engage in rehabilitation with the sports therapist, in physical and cardiorespiratory conditioning with the physical trainer, and to have the appropriate support from other team members (as nutritionists, psychologists, among others). This working dynamics reflect the coordinated action made possible by the existence of a hired medical staff dedicated to professional athletes. This context allows these athletes to concentrate on the planned program, which help them to return to the sport as quickly as possible. The routine of the rehabilitation program for an Olympic level athlete (which includes high-level amateur athlete) is influenced by the type and severity of the injury and its consequences for sport performance. During the treatment of the injured athlete, the sports therapist should tie the rehabilitation program with a program of physical and cardiorespiratory conditioning to prevent some loss of the athlete's fitness level. In addition, the sports therapist's presence during training is necessary to identify the demand imposed on the athlete's musculoskeletal system and to analyze possible repercussions for the process of injury recovery. At a specific moment, determined by all professionals involved in the rehabilitation process (i.e., sports therapist, physical trainer, and physician), the athlete may be allowed to take part in the whole training regime or just part of it. Physical therapy intervention may be implemented to maintain treatment gains and to reinsert the athlete into a return to competition/prevention program. Thus, the available organizational/logistical structure allows all the team professionals to discuss the demand to be imposed on the athlete, in order to provide the necessary training overload without increasing injury susceptibility.

Some well-structured amateur athletes who participate in Olympic events may receive similar medical attention as professional athletes, if they have sufficient funding to set up or have access to an integrated medical team. However, one of the main differences between amateur and professional athletes is the possibility of losing a continuing source of income (sponsorship) and not receiving proper care after the Olympic event, especially in case of a disabling injury. Professional athletes, who are under long contracts, know that even after a severe injury, which could lead to their removal from competitions, they will still receive adequate treatment and participate in specific programs to allow return to sports. In some cases, the professional athlete, together with the medical team, may even decide to continue to compete after a nondisabling injury. This decision is based on the expectation and assurance that he or she will receive post-event attention. On the other hand, the occurrence of a disabling injury during competition in some nonprofessional athletes may result in loss of sponsorships and jeopardize their access to adequate medical assistance after the event. This process can alter the athlete's expectations and the relationship with the sport therapist. Therefore, professional athletes have a more stable career and may be willing to take some risk during Olympic Games.

Working with amateur athletes

The care to the amateur athlete provided by a sports therapist is clearly based on the same theoretical considerations that guide the clinical reasoning presented (founded on the relationship between demand and capacity). The approach to this athlete may also include rehabilitation, functional return, and injury prevention. However, the opportunities for emergency care and early rehabilitation for this athlete are less frequently available. Another frequent limitation is that, depending on the amount of funding the amateur athlete can obtain (i.e., personal or sponsorships), he or she may not be able to organize a coordinated team to provide proper care. Thus, the care providers, including the sports therapist, may not be able to establish a coordinated intervention/prevention program to address the athlete's needs. For example, if there is no physical trainer on the team assembled by the amateur athlete, the cardiorespiratory work may be inappropriate for the return to competition planned by the sports therapist. In addition, the selected members of the medical team of the amateur athlete may not have adequate knowledge of the sport (or the athletic demand) as they are frequently hired through third-party referrals or their contributions are dependent upon private consulting, sometimes available from the athlete's health plan.

In general, the lack of continuous professional monitoring of the athlete's health can lead the amateur athlete to seek care only when an injury has reached an advanced stage, after trying nonoriented treatment and self-medication. In this last case, symptoms may be masked by the medication. This facilitates a painless sport practice, which may, in turn, aggravate the injury. During rehabilitation and functional return of the amateur athlete, clinical decisions on evolution and release for sport practice highly depend on the stage of injury at the moment the athlete sought treatment. It also depends on the extent of the athlete's involvement in the treatment and on the time available for rehabilitation, since the amateur athletes dedicate simultaneously to their sport activity and to their occupation, while for professionals, the sport is their occupation. In addition to less time for daily dedication to sport, some amateur athletes may not follow therapeutic recommendations and may return to activity before the sports therapist thinks they are ready, which harms the return of the athlete to his or her preinjury level of performance. The early return to sport can also occur with professional athlete, but this is mainly due to pressure from coaches and sponsors.

In contrast to Olympic level athletes, amateur athletes often are not involved in controlled physical preparation and training. The training demand is not administrated by a health care team, which may result in excessive or decreased loading for the musculoskeletal system. Specifically, the lack of scientifically coordinated and planned training may result in inappropriate loading of joints or biological tissues. In cases in which the athlete imposes excessive overload to the musculoskeletal system, the demand exceeds the adaptation capability (i.e., unfavorable demand/capacity relation), performance decreases, and injury may occur. In cases in which the athlete imposes an insufficient and less frequent loading, the system's capability decreases. They often increase the level of training abruptly near competition periods, which may constitute a temporary excessive overload to the musculoskeletal system. A clear example of this last case is when the amateur athletes take part only in the practice of the sport, without working on their neuromusculoskeletal resources (e.g., strength training) that optimizes the system capacity to deal with the stress demands of the sport.

Regardless of the difficulties of the amateur athletes' care, some of these athletes are aware of the determinants of performance, injury occurrence and rehabilitation, and have adequate financial support provided by sponsors. Athletes with this profile often have higher expectations related to performance. Thus, they require professional monitoring and are explicitly concerned with performance evolution. Although they have to partition their time between the sport and their professional activity, they are able to have sports therapy care before the occurrence of painful conditions and in the early stages of an injury. This permits the sport therapist to plan and give appropriate orientation for prevention and treatment.

Besides the difference involved in general context related to athletes' status (professional vs. amateur) previously discussed, the sports therapist's attention to these athletes depends on the structure involved in each particular sports organization. While some sports associations have administrative and economic structures that allow an appropriate organization for a sports medicine team, others do not. In order to exemplify the influence of sports structure on the sports therapist work, the Brazilian volleyball and soccer contexts are presented. However, it is important to understand that there are no clear-cut differences between the care of high-level amateurs and professionals. Many amateurs have, early on, minimal support but as they improve in their sport and begin to make Olympic standard, they obtain, through sponsorship and often government funding, similar care to professional athletes. This greater level of funding will depend on the ability of the amateur and his or her support team to find sources of funding support. The possibility of support increases if the athlete has the potential to "finish in the medals." The professional

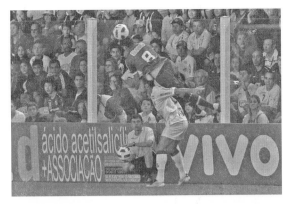
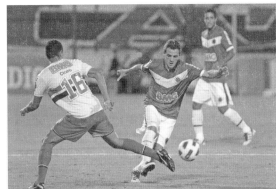
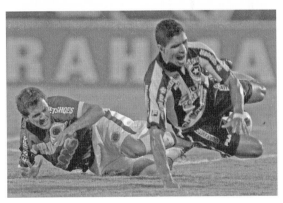
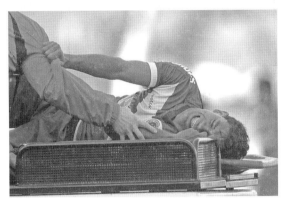

Figure 8.1 Football (soccer)—played by professionals and amateurs in Brazil (Reprinted with permission from the Cruzeiro Esporte Clube)

on the other hand can often afford to pay for the support himself or herself or may expect a higher level of support in return for competing for his or her country.

Examples of the Brazilian sports therapist's role in football (soccer) and volleyball

In a global context, (soccer) football and volleyball are the most popular sports in Brazil, with approximately 30 million and 15 million participants, respectively (Figures 8.1 and 8.2). Soccer and volleyball popularity in Brazil is evidenced by the high frequency of amateur athletes' participation in private organizations, such as clubs, private sports arenas, and public arenas, often located in under-

privileged communities. Therefore, many talented players are discovered in these settings. In addition to this great popularity, volley and soccer receive much attention from sports media and much of the financial investment is directed to these sports in Brazil. This large financial investment makes possible the formation of appropriate staff having exclusive dedication to the professional athlete as well as appropriate physical and administrative structures. The great popularity of these organizations in Brazil and the existence of both professional and amateur structures make football (soccer) and volleyball good examples for the sports therapy practice. In addition, differences in the organizational structures of these organizations and in the socioeconomic level of their participants allow a better understanding of the expectations of the athletes.

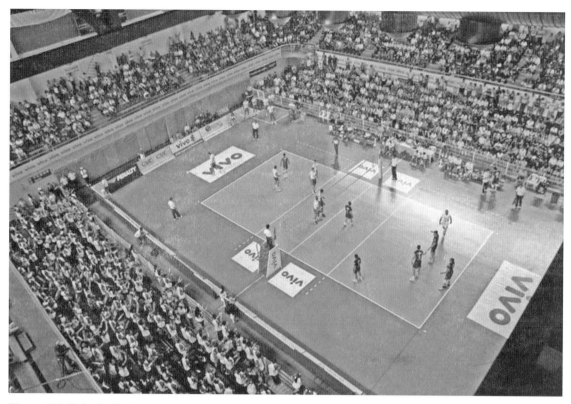

Figure 8.2 Volleyball—played by professionals and amateurs in Brazil (Reproduced with permission from the Minas Tênis Clube, 2010—Photographer Orlando Bento)

Sports therapy approach for both volleyball and football (soccer) professional athletes depends on the player's category, since the clinical process of decision making must consider the athlete's preparation, physical condition, and the competition agenda. This permits the sports therapist to analyze the overload and recovery of the athlete. In volleyball, for instance, there are four categories, according to the player technical level or age:

1 The adult athlete who is member of the Brazilian team who has a short preseason period for an adequate preparation. This athlete frequently has intermediary resting periods of just 1 week between seasons in the Brazilian team and regional seasons of his or her club.

2 The adult athlete of a club, who takes part in an appropriate preseason that lasts around 3 months and who participates in small tournaments

as a preparation for the national championship (Superliga).

3 The young athlete (talent), who is part of the youth Brazilian team and (due to his or her distinguished performance) is also a member of the adult team of a club.

4 The amateur athlete, who competes in competitions with a high school or college team or in a nonprofessional sport or social club.

The Brazilian team that participates in Olympic events can be composed of athletes from distinct categories and clubs (except from category four). Consequently, the sports therapist may deal with athletes who have not been subjected to a preventive program, with those who come from an intense rhythm of different competitions and athletes who participate in adequate preseason preparations.

In football (soccer), a similar process can be observed. Football (soccer) athletes are part of diverse categories, varying from professional players on national and international clubs to young athletes (talents) in these clubs to nonfederated amateur athletes. The Brazilian Olympic team consists of professional athletes younger than 23 years who play on national and international teams. Due to their diverse origins, these athletes may have been subjected to distinct training and rehabilitation demands over their competition seasons. These different demands can influence the athletes' performance and susceptibility to injury.

Considering the variety of the athletes from official volleyball and football (soccer) teams, sports therapists who work on Olympic teams must plan the preventive and rehabilitative activities of each athlete (on an individual basis), considering the athlete's history related to demands of previous competitions, intensity of technical and tactical training sessions, injury occurrence, and the capacity of the athlete's musculoskeletal system. Frequently, lack of information about these factors and the short period of preparation prevent the implementation of effective individual strategies.

The work of the sports therapist, both in volleyball and football (soccer), is influenced by the specific context of the setting in which the work is conducted. Football (soccer) in Brazil, for example, comprises 800 professional clubs, with 11,000 federated athletes and 13,000 amateur teams. The organizational structure of each of these clubs and thus the work conditions for the athletes, sports therapist, and other medical team members may vary. Regarding the professional teams of both organizations, the team staff, in general, communicates about the procedures used in the rehabilitation process, and the athlete is informed about his or her condition. These dynamics create coresponsibility for all individuals involved, mainly for the athlete. In this context, the athlete has a more active participation in the rehabilitation process, allowing adjustments in the athlete's expectations relative to recovery and return to training and competition. A process of coparticipation should determine the rehabilitation and training routines and predictions on the athlete's return to competition. Due to the professional support, the athlete and the entire staff of the team expect the earliest possible return to the sport practice, which often brings more dis-

advantages than advantages. Pressure for return to competition may lead to a premature reinsertion of the athlete into training sessions and competition, within an insufficient time for appropriate repair of the injured tissue. Premature return may lead to a loss in performance or to injury recurrence, as the athlete has not fully recovered. Hence, dealing with the anxiety of the athlete and other members of the team staff, related to treatment duration, is a challenge for the sports therapist involved with professional teams, both in volleyball and football (soccer).

At the beginning of a season, the sports therapist who works with professional athletes has the opportunity to evaluate the players, going over their injury history or sequelae due to incomplete rehabilitation. After an initial assessment, a preventive program is established. For this program to be effective, the sports therapist must ensure that the exercises/interventions will be included in the athletes' routine, even during competitions and travel. Therefore, the sports therapist who works with volleyball and football (soccer) professionals has the opportunity to act at various levels. Furthermore, there is an opportunity to obtain reliable contributions from other professionals in the planning and execution of programs of prevention, treatment, and return to activity.

Unlike the professional athlete, the amateur athlete, mainly in Brazilian football (soccer), is rarely exposed to a program focused on injury prevention, because of the lack of adequate support. Thus, in addition to not receiving appropriate immediate/emergency treatment, these athletes are unprepared to avoid the occurrence and recurrence of injuries. In volleyball, some amateur athletes are part of minimally developed organizations, within social clubs and schools. Therefore, these athletes receive minimal medical monitoring. However, in this context, the sports therapist acts only at the rehabilitation level, with minimal or no opportunity to implement prevention programs or to provide adequate care for return to competition.

The amateur athlete is often not subjected to the same pressures that the professional athlete receives from sponsors and coaches, although he or she is under pressure to succeed and receive the rewards that will follow from that success. Furthermore, there are not as many competitions for amateurs to be involved in. These characteristics may allow for a longer period of rehabilitation, which allows appropriate tissue recovery. However, return to activity is more difficult since the sports therapist often cannot monitor or control the training load of the amateur athlete. Hence, even with a longer time for rehabilitation, the care given to this athlete is often inadequate and may result in an excessively prolonged and inefficient return to activity.

The existence of well-developed, professional and amateur organizations in Brazilian volleyball and football (soccer) permits one to make a rich analysis of the sports therapist's work and of the expectations and anxieties of the athletes. The realities of professionals and amateurs of these organizations are so different that in many sports, only professional athletes have an opportunity to participate in the Olympic Games. However, other sports, such as fencing or rowing, whose organizational structures are less developed and do not have professional leagues, allow amateur athletes to achieve performance levels sufficient to participate in Olympic Games. Even with a less-developed organizational structure, in these sports, the amateur athletes often have the support of an advanced team of health care professionals. This context leads to another situation: the presence of nonofficial sports therapists and trainers at Olympic events. The next section will present this theme and discuss the work of the sports therapist during Olympic events.

Official versus private therapist working with Olympic athletes

During competitions, official (belonging to the sports medicine team) and private (brought by athletes) sports therapists may have the opportunity to provide care to athletes. These sport therapists have different roles and abilities, as their knowledge of the athlete and sport may vary. This atypical situation may cause some discomfort in the relationship between the athlete and the official sport therapist and, sometimes, may constrain the contribution of both therapists to the athlete's well-being. The configuration of the members of an Olympic delegation responsible for the care of athletes during Olympic events depends on a norm established by the IOC. The IOC establishes that the maximum number of health care professionals of a given country allowed in the games should be 4% in relation to the number of athletes of that delegation. The smaller the number of athletes attending the games, the more difficult is the distribution of these professionals among the various areas, such as medicine, physical therapy, and psychology. In the Olympic Games, the delegation's sports therapists, independently of their expertise, are responsible for the emergency care and treatment of injuries of the athletes of all sport modalities. Thus, official sports therapists must have technical knowledge to treat the elite athlete and know about the specificities of each sport. The sports therapist must also know the rules about the emergency care in each sport, the use of equipments, and doping. In parallel to the official sports therapists, private therapists are selected and sponsored by the athletes themselves. As such, they are commonly not part of the country's "official" team. Despite their proper knowledge of the athletes and the specific sport, they are commonly not able to have full access to the athlete or have the chance to help the medical team to make decisions about the athlete's practice/performance condition.

In the Olympic context, there is the need to select a sports therapist team that is prepared to deal with the particularities of several different sports. This may not be the reality of all therapists working in Olympic events. In Brazil, for example, sports therapists tend to specialize in a given sport and may not have enough knowledge to treat athletes in other sports. Rarely, an official sports therapist has the specific knowledge of the demands and rules of several sports in which the country participates. Due to the requirements of having specialized and, at the same time, broad enough knowledge to attend to different sports, selecting professionals with these qualities to compose the Olympic medical team may be a great challenge to any country's Olympic committee.

With the objective to minimize possible interferences in the performance of teams and elite athletes, sports therapists who are part of the medical staff of these teams or athletes are frequently incorporated into the country's Olympic delegation. The advantage of this procedure is the possibility of continuity with the work in progress and the greater familiarity of the sports therapist with the rules and requirements of the sport. However, the contribution of these sports therapists may be restricted, as the final decision about the athlete's treatment or prevention work is, frequently, centered in the official head sports therapist, who may have different opinion about the planned interventions.

Some professional athletes with better financial means may allow the presence of their private sports therapist during the Olympic Games. This individual's presence may give the athlete the comfort of knowing that he or she may receive care from the professional who has followed him or her during the preparation period and know his or her characteristics and needs. During the Olympic Games, the role of the private therapist is to contribute to the athlete's recovery during the intervals between games or competitions. However, private therapists commonly do not have access to the Olympic Village except as visitors and the care provided to the athlete is frequently done at an outside location (e.g., a hotel) and in a concealed manner. The athlete may also have difficulty receiving private medical care, as there are regulations about the circulation of people inside the Olympic Village. In addition to this restriction, some Olympic committees (e.g., the Brazilian Olympic Committee) do not officially support the participation of private therapists during the Olympic Games, as differences in care provided between official and private sports therapists may cause more harm than benefits, as well as be disruptive to the team concept they are trying to build. Therefore, despite the possible benefits that the presence of private sports therapists may bring to the individual athlete, the delegation's officials often do not see this situation with approval.

Professional high-level athletes frequently bring their private therapists to the Olympic Games. Similarly, many national teams (e.g., basketball, volleyball, and football/soccer) include their own sports therapist as part of their own Olympic delegation. The main problem resides in the care sometimes provided to amateur athletes or low-profile teams. In these cases, the athletes depend solely on the care provided by official medical team, since they do not have enough financial resources to afford their own therapists. The lack of specific knowledge of the sport and the athletes' conditions and characteristics may reduce the efficiency of the care provided and jeopardize their performance. In Brazil, amateur athletes rarely have proper training infrastructure that help them to attain Olympic standards. Those who manage to integrate the country's Olympic team must rely on official sports therapists during competition. In this sense, the process of selecting official therapists must always consider the sports therapist's knowledge of the different requirements and demands of the several sports, in which they will be asked to provide care.

References

Akeson, W.H., Woo, S.L.Y. & Amiel, D. (1984) The chemical basis of tissue repair. In: L.Y. Hunter & F.J. Funk (eds) *Rehabilitation of the Injured Knee*, Mosby, St. Louis, MO.

Athanasopoulos, S., Kapreli, E., Tsakoniti, A., Karatsolis, K., Diamantopoulos, K., Kalampakas, K., Pyrros, D.G., Parisis, C. & Strimpakos, N. (2007) The 2004 Olympic Games: physiotherapy services in the Olympic Village polyclinic. *British Journal of Sports Medicine*, 41, 603–609.

Badekas, T., Papadakis, S.A., Vergados, N., Galanakos, S.P., Siapkara, A., Forgrave, M., Romansky, N., Mirones, S., Trnka, H.J. & Delmi, M. (2009) Foot and ankle injuries during the Athens 2004 Olympic Games. *Journal of Foot and Ankle Research*, 2(9), 1–8.

Burke, L. (1995) Practical issues in nutrition for athletes. *Journal of Sports Science*, 13, S83–S90.

Butler, R.J., Crowell, H.P. & Davis, I.M. (2003) Lower extremity stiffness: implications for performance and injury. *Clinical Biomechanics (Bristol, Avon)*, 18(6), 511–517.

Elphinston, J. & Hardman, S.L. (2006) Effect of an integrated functional stability program on injury rates in an international netball squad. *Journal of Science and Medicine and Sports* 9, 169–176.

Fonseca, S.T., Ocarino, J.M., Silva, P.L.P. & Aquino, C.F. (2007) Integration of stresses and their relationship to the kinetic chain. In: D.J. Magee, J.E. Zachazewski & W.S. Quillen (eds) *Scientific Foundations and Principles of Practice in Musculoskeletal Rehabilitation*, Saunders, St. Louis, MO.

Fonseca, S.T., Souza, T.R., Ocarino, J.M., Gonçalves, G.P. & Bittencourt, F.N. (2010) Applied biomechanics of soccer. In D.J. Magee, J.E. Zachazewski & W.S. Quillen (eds) *Athletic and Sport Issues in Musculoskeletal Rehabilitation*, Saunders, St. Louis, MO.

Fonseca, S.T., Holt, K.G., Fetters, L. & Saltzman, E. (2004) Dynamic resources used in ambulation by children with spastic hemiplegic cerebral palsy: relationship to kinematics, energetics, and asymmetries. *Physical Therapy*, 84(4), 344–354; discussion 355–358.

Garrett, W.E. Jr., Safran, M.R., Seaber, A.V. *et al.* (1987) Biomechanical comparison of stimulated and non-stimulated skeletal muscle pulled to failure. *American Journal of Sports Medicine*, 15(5), 448–454.

Goforth, M., Almquist, J., Matney, M., Abdenour, T.E., Kyle, J., Leaman, J. & Montgomery, S. (2007) Understanding organization structures of the college, university, high school, clinical, and professional settings. *Clinics in Sports Medicine*, 26(2), 201–226.

Huijing, P.A. & Jaspers, R.T. (2005) Adaptation of muscle size and myofascial force transmission: a review and some new experimental results. *Scandinavian Journal of Medicine and Science Sports*, 15, 349–380.

Junge, A., Engebretsen, L., Alonso, J.M., Renstro, P., Mountjoy, M., Aubry, M. & Dvorak, J. (2008) Injury surveillance in multi-sport events: the International Olympic Committee approach. *British Journal of Sports Medicine*, 42, 413–421.

Junge, A., Engebretsen, L., Mountjoy, M.L., Alonso, J.M., Renström, P.A.F.H., Aubry, M.J. & Dvorak, J. (2009) Sports injuries during the summer Olympic Games 2008. *American Journal of Sports Medicine*, 37, 2165–2172.

Michaud, T.C. (1993) Abnormal motion during the gait cycle. In: T.C. Michaud (ed) *Foot Orthoses and Other Forms of Conservative Foot Care*, Williams & Wilkins, Baltimore, MD.

Myers, T.W. (2009) *Anatomy Trains: Myofascial Meridians for Manual and Movement Therapists*, 2nd edn, Churchill Livingstone Elsevier, Edinburgh.

Nosfinger, C.C. (2007) Negotiating contractual relationship. *Clinics in Sports Medicine*, 26(2), 193–199.

Pensgaard, A.M. & Ursin, H. (1998) Stress, control, and coping in elite athletes. *Scandinavian Journal of Medicine and Science in Sports*, 8(3), 183–189.

Silva, A.A., Bittencourt, N.F.N., Mendonça, L.M., Tirado, M.G., Sampaio, R.F. & Fonseca, S. (2011) Analysis of the profile, areas of action and abilities of Brazilian sports physical therapists working with soccer and volleyball. *Brazilian Journal of Physical Therapy*, 15(3), 219–226.

Thelwell, R.C., Weston, N.J., Greenlees, I.A. & Hutchings, N.V. (2008) Stressors in elite sport: a coach perspective. *Journal of Sports Science*, 26(9), 905–918.

Vleeming, A., Pool-Goudzwaard, A.L., Stoeckart, R. *et al.* (1995) The posterior layer of the thoracolumbar fascia—its function in load transfer from spine to legs. *Spine*, 20(7), 753–758.

Wetterhall, S.F., Coulombier, D.M., Herndon, J.M., Zaza, S. & Cantwell, J.D. (1998) Medical care delivery at the 1996 Olympic Games. *Journal of the American Medical Association*, 279, 1463–1468.

Zajac, F.E., Neptune, R.R. & Kautz, S.A. (2002) Biomechanics and muscle coordination of human walking. Part I: Introduction to concepts, power transfer, dynamics and simulations. *Gait Posture*, 16, 215–232.

Chapter 9

To compete or not to compete following injury during Olympic events

Tony Ward

Australian Institute of Sport, Belconnen, ACT, Australia

Introduction

The return to competition scenario could be described as a routine responsibility of the sports medicine professional working with the team or an individual athlete within the elite sporting arena. As required with the management of each elite athlete's injury, there will be the considerations of when and how to return the athlete to his or her normal training and competition loads. It is important to acknowledge that the conditions for an athlete's return to competition and training vary greatly, even for those who seem to be seen in very similar circumstances or to have an identical injury diagnosis. This routine obligation also becomes the first and ultimate question on the lips of every athlete, coach, or team manager—when will the athlete be able to compete (or train) again?

> For athletes, the Olympics are the ultimate test of their worth.
>
> Mary Lou Retton
> USA gymnast 1984 summer Olympic Games
> http://quotations.about.com/od/sportsquotes/a/olympics2.htm

Experiences gained from working with an elite group of athletes have led the author to recognize that having a decision-making process that is both effective and direct is paramount for the success of return to competition assessments (Figure 9.1). The return to competition dilemma and decision is never greater than one that surrounds an Olympic athlete at the games as this is commonly the pinnacle sporting event in many athletes' careers.

An injury prior to or during the Olympic Games can be a devastating experience not only for the athlete but also for all parties involved, including the coach, teammates, medical staff, team officials, and families. Associated with the injury is the pressure that is then placed on the immediate medical staff's decision for the athlete to compete or not to compete. Within major competitions such as the Olympic Games, this critical decision can unfortunately become distorted in its processing and amplified in importance. However, as the sports medicine professional in charge of the athlete, one cannot lose sight of the basic ideal and responsibility that establishes the foundation of the decision-making process: the overall safety of the athletes.

General return to competition guidelines were formally described in 2002 through the formation of a team physicians consensus statement. This statement essentially outlined four factors that

---

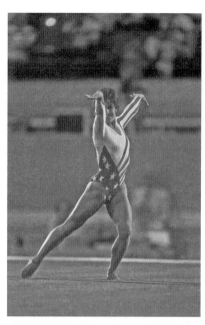

Figure 9.1 Sound medical and therapeutic decisions are key considerations in the return of an injured athlete to competition at elite events such as the Olympic Games (Photo courtesy of the International Olympic Committee)

appeared mandatory when returning athletes back to competing in their sport (Herring *et al.* 2002):
1 Safety of the athlete.
2 Potential risk to the safety of other athletes.
3 Functional capabilities of the athlete.
4 Functional requirements of the athlete's sport.

It is important to highlight that the actual requirements in the decision-making process at an elite level of sport go beyond these basic guidelines. This chapter will outline a number of specific decision-making requirements through the experiences of an Olympic sports physiotherapist, in addressing the issue of athlete participation following injury (Figure 9.2).

Understanding aspects in the clinical decision-making process

---

First, one needs to be sensitive to and understand the actual decision-making processes that are

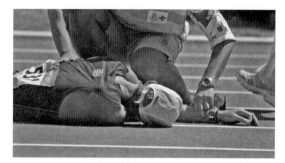

Figure 9.2 Medical personnel checking vital signs of athlete who has collapsed following event. Critical evaluative and decision-making skills are vital in order for the sports therapist to provide the best care and advice possible to the athlete relative to competition after injury or illness

evoked when one is required to address the question of an athlete's return to sport. This can be best described in terms of the clinician's skill and ability in clinical reasoning.

What is clinical reasoning?

In general terms, clinical reasoning can be described as the thinking and decision-making processes that clinicians use to arrive at a decision in the clinical practice. It incorporates how one generates and evaluates ideas or solves problems in an accurate and thoughtful process. Effective clinical reasoning can enable the clinician to respond to the athlete's concerns and questions and give confidence to the athlete and coach regarding the athlete's readiness to return to sport.

Clinical reasoning has been described as having three core elements (Higgs *et al.* 2008):
1 **Cognition**: the mental action or process of thought or acquiring knowledge and understanding through thought, experience, and the senses.
2 **Metacognition**: the knowledge and awareness of one's own thinking processes and strategies, including the ability to evaluate and regulate these processes.
3 **Knowledge**: the information and skills acquired through experience or education, this being one's theoretical or practical understanding of a subject.

Within these three core elements, knowledge has been the one element described as the likely key to one's clinical reasoning skills. More importantly, it is in one's ability to organize this knowledge base that improves the skills of clinical reasoning and separates the novice and expert clinicians.

Novice problem solvers often tend to be more superficial in their knowledge leading to fragmentation of their ideas; and they often appear more literal, often without understanding the consequences of their actions or they are likely to get caught by the hidden issues that are missed.

In comparison, an expert is commonly able to question the situation in a succinct fashion with meaningful purpose. It can also be said that the expert may be better at evaluating the situation and interpreting clinical examinations when required. Experts in clinical reasoning also have an ability to focus on any unusual aspects of the problems.

So how does one become an expert in clinical reasoning? The key elements to developing expert clinical reasoning skills are time and experience. This should be augmented by taking an active role in the decisions regarding an athlete's injury, treatment, and rehabilitation. Continually challenging the way one thinks in terms of problem solving associated with an athlete's injury, care and rehabilitation can also enhance the skills of clinical reasoning.

Why is good clinical reasoning so important?

Having good clinical reasoning skills allows the clinician to repetitively make the best decision for athletes being cared for no matter what the injury or situation. This consistency in judgment can give the athlete a high degree of confidence in advice rendered by the sports therapist and the therapist's ability to help the athlete make the best decision regarding his or her health and ability to return to competition.

It is important to remember that each decision is very specific both to the sporting environment and the individual athlete involved and therefore should be treated as such. Using appropriate and effective clinical reasoning skills prevents the sports therapist from following a "recipe" approach toward managing athlete injuries, and more importantly their rehabilitation and decision regarding return to sport during the games.

In each specific case, an individualized plan should be developed, referring to a basic checklist of an athlete's readiness to return to sport. This checklist should include but not be restricted to aspects such as those described by Brukner and Khan (2007):

• Sufficient time to allow for adequate soft tissue healing within the expected constraints of an acute injury process or current state of a chronic injury.
• No functional deficits present at the time of returning to sport.
• No joint instability or persistent swelling.
• Adequate strength and endurance.
• Psychological readiness of the athlete.
• Approval of the coach.
• Risk of reinjury or injury to either themselves or others is minimal.

However, the use of a "recipe," compared with an individualized plan for each athlete's particular injury, is fraught with dangers. Due to the pressures of competing at an Olympic Games, a return to sport assessment should be based on the clinician's highly skilled assessment and judgment, individualized to the specific situation. This utilizes the best clinical reasoning process through the clinician's experience and enables an athlete to have a high degree of confidence in the clinician's judgment (Figure 9.3).

The role of the sports physiotherapist in relationship to physicians and other medical staff

Just as important as the decision of when to return the athlete to activity is the question of who sits in the ultimate position to make the decision regarding an injured athlete's return to sport. The decision-making role of a sports physiotherapist varies relative to the specific timing of the event. This can differ depending on whether the injury has occurred within competition or is identified pre- or post-event. The sports physiotherapist's involvement in an athlete's overall treatment or

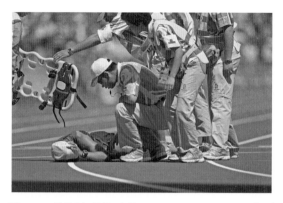

Figure 9.3 Multidisciplinary emergency medical team responds to care for injured athletes at summer games. Highly skilled assessment and judgment is critical in emergency care situations (Photo courtesy of the International Olympic Committee)

rehabilitation programming is usually very high, as is the understanding of an athlete's readiness to compete. However, the actual responsibility for the decision of an athlete's return to sport will inevitably vary depending upon the clinician's sports experience and the total dynamics of each sports medicine team.

A hierarchal medical system is in place in most sporting organizations, teams, or clubs. Within the elite sporting arena or event such as the Olympics, it is usually acknowledged that the senior physician for a team has the final say regarding an athlete's return to competition. The precise outline of the decision-making hierarchy must be made early within the medical team setup and duly followed through for it to be effective. However, because there is often a limitation in medical staff numbers, the roles and responsibilities of the staff members may vary. With an increased responsibility, the sports therapist may have a greater role within the event than outside of the event during the games. The utilization of valuable advice from all members of the medical staff should be utilized to the fullest potential when the return to compete question is posed. To this end, it is apparent that the final decision to compete in the elite sporting arena is improved when there is a collaboration of thoughts from an experienced multidisciplinary sports medicine team or network.

It is evident that the final decision regarding whether to continue to participate in the games as a specific result of an injury should not be left up to either a coach or team administrator. In these situations, any risk of a conflict of interest, real or perceived, must be avoided. Coaches and administrators are also often limited in their total understanding of the injury or related risks of returning to competition. Hence, effective communication and team policy regarding decisions concerning the return to compete process must be established early. This is not only to maintain a good coach and medical staff relationship but also to improve the effectiveness of setting up an appropriate decision-making chain of command within the full team or squad.

The roles and responsibility of the sports therapist within this context may differ considerably during international competition or tours. The differences in actual roles and responsibility are most often due to the therapist's position as either the sole medical provider accompanying a team or as a member of a larger medical team. Within each of these positions, responsibilities differ greatly. However, the importance of having an accurate and established line of decision making remains constant from a basic domestic tour within a country to the high-pressured competition of an Olympic Games.

To firmly establish the role of the sports physiotherapist or medical professional regarding the athlete's return to competition process, the following criteria are essential:
• Establishing the appropriate working communication channels between all medical staff, team officials, coaches, administrators, and athletes.
• Taking an active role in the decision-making process when required.
• Understanding the process and continuing to develop one's skills and experience.
• Avoiding overstepping one's position or responsibility; however, one should also be sufficiently confident to express one's professional opinions when it is called for.

If communication is established in the correct way, it can be invaluable for the athlete's return to sport decision. At some stage in the career of any sports therapist, the decision will fall squarely on his/her shoulders. Experience, communication, and clinical reasoning skills will allow the sports therapist to effectively meet the challenge he or she faces.

The process of making a return to sport decision

In some circumstances, the leading question will not be when can the athlete return to competition or training, but rather can an athlete physically return or not? Obviously, if the medical response is no, then the decision to return to activity goes no further. However, in the showground of sport, there are a significant number of components that need to be taken into consideration before the ultimate decision to compete or not is made. This decision relates highly to the specific sporting situation, and therefore can vary considerably even for similar injuries due to the environment or circumstance of the competition. One must be aware that the complexities of the individual sporting situations can make assessment more difficult due to the increased factors that need to be considered (Table 9.1). This is exactly why the environment of an Olympic Games can distort some possibilities in the decision-making process.

A clinician's decision can be centered on acute management of injuries, the things that would be considered as being specific to on-field manage- ment guidelines. They may also be based on injury management procedures prior to or following competition as part of daily treatment responsibilities. For example, there has been substantial literature written on management of concussion injuries during sport including formal guidelines, but at the same time, the mandatory recovery periods have changed so that each case is treated individually and is very much symptom related.

As mentioned previously, expert sports physiotherapists handle these situations well, whereas less experienced therapists need greater understanding and clinical reasoning to determine when the athlete can return to activity, to the point where cues through a model approach may be beneficial. Again, it needs to be emphasized that when looking at specific models, one should not see them as a recipe approach, rather as guidelines to help develop skills in one's clinical reasoning.

Creighton *et al.* (2010) developed an appropriate model of return to play guidelines. They proposed a three-step diagram highlighting the need to consider all components within the decision-making process (Table 9.2). Their proposal was an attempt to reduce controversy and improve progression when deciding the appropriate course of action.

If these components are added to those from the 2002 consensus guidelines presented earlier in this chapter, a relatively robust outline is provided. However, each situation still needs to be assessed

Table 9.1 Possible complexities in the return to sport decisions

	Lower Complexity	**Higher Complexity**
Sporting situation	• Training • General competition • Domestic season	• Selection trials • World championships • Olympic Games
Season timing	• Start of season • Including preseason • Heats	• End of season • Including final series • Playoffs or final
Squad	• Team competition with player reserves • Team sports with different playing positions	• Individual competition • Specific team events without reserves
Injury timing	• Post-event • Pre-event with allowance for adequate treatment	• In competition injuries • Pre-event with limited treatment time
Injury type	• Minor injury • Chronic ongoing injury • Limited performance issue	• Major injury • Acute and competition ending • Performance affected

Table 9.2 Return to play guidelines

Evaluation of Health	Participation Risk	Decision Modification
• Athlete demographics	• Type of sport (contact vs. noncontact)	• Time of season
• Symptoms	• Playing position of athlete	• Pressure from athlete
• History, signs, symptoms	• Limb dominance vs. side injured	• External pressure from others
• Diagnostic and clinical tests	• Competition level	• Ability to mask injury (medical)
• Psychological state	• Ability to protect injury	• Conflict of interest and risk of
• Seriousness of initial injury		litigation

Data from Creighton *et al.* (2010).

separately and therefore needs to consider all factors, such as the status or importance of the event. These factors will always vary within events such as a country's domestic elite competition, an international event, a world championship, or an Olympic Games. This remains extremely important when consideration of winning at one level of competition may lead to further progression in elite competitive events all the way to the Olympics and possibly to an Olympic medal. Again, it is the sports medicine professional's role to be aware of all aspects in their decision-making process including the significant team dynamics such as the following:

• Importance of the athlete within the team group.
• Will the athlete make a valuable contribution to the team/game if he or she returns?
• Will there be more games, following this one?
• Does the athlete understand the full risks of competing with the injury?

During discussions about an athlete's readiness to return to competition or training, there is obviously a significant focus on the athlete's functional capability. With this specific focus, the athlete's state of mind, which is just as critical as his/her physical function, may unfortunately not be considered sufficiently when considering return to sport. Clinical decision making must take into consideration the fact that there is a strong link between both psychological and functional states to an athlete's actual performance. This might then help answer the question of whether or not the athlete is being pushed into competition too early prior to an absolute resolution of their injuries or are they fully prepared for the rigors of elite sport. One must remember that the decision should consider the collective input of all members of the sports medicine and coaching staff available.

For example, Verrall *et al.* (2006) made reference to this collective decision making in a study that assessed player performance following return to sport after hamstring muscle strains. Their 2-year study of playing performance after hamstring injuries in Australian Rules Football (AFL) found that the coach rated player performance (ranked between 1 and 10) dropped significantly within the athlete's first two games back into competition (Figure 9.4).

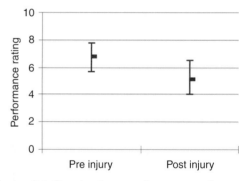

Figure 9.4 Coach–player performance ratings pre- and postinjury. Thirteen athletes had hamstring injuries and the required player ratings were available. Mean player performance rating for the entire season in which the player was injured was 6.9. Mean rating for the two games prior to injury was 6.8 as opposed to 5.4 for the two games after returning to sport. Player performance rating was significantly lower ($p < 0.001$) immediately on return to sport when compared with ratings for the entire season, and when compared with rating from the two games prior to injury ($p < 0.001$) (Data from Verrall *et al.* 2006)

This poses two questions. First, were these athletes in fact returning to sport too early? And, second, was this an isolated factor to an AFL athlete and/or hamstring injuries or was it a more common occurrence association across a wider variety of sports and athlete injuries? If it is indeed a common event across sports and injuries, it highlights the essential fact that athlete's readiness to return to elite competition must include accessing their psychological preparation.

Impact of decision on team performance or an individual athlete's career

An overall balance must be struck between an athlete's rapid return to sport and reducing his or her risk of injury recurrence. What is the balance between risk of further and possibly more serious/permanent injury and the gain of victory/performance? To answer this, a critical question must be asked by everyone, which is at what stage does an athlete's injury risk become acceptable (Figure 9.5).

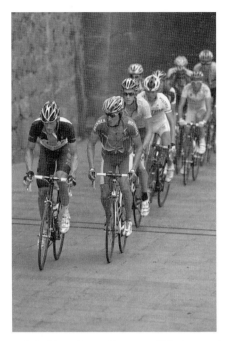

Figure 9.5 Olympic cyclists on difficult terrain requiring them to conquer "pain" associated with required effort for Olympic performance and excellence (Photo courtesy of the International Olympic Committee)

> Pain is temporary. It may last a minute, an hour, a day, or a year, but eventually it will subside and something else will take its place. If I quit, however it will last forever
>
> Lance Armstrong
> Cycling Champion
> http://gymnastics.about.com/u/ua/
> gettingstarted/InspirationalQuotes.01.htm

Working with elite athletes can be a difficult scenario as an athlete's temperament and passion to perform can conflict with the overall team focus, especially if there is any concern regarding an athlete's ongoing performance due to injury. Although there is an underlying responsibility to the athlete and his or her imminent career, it must also be noted that there is a greater duty of responsibility to the team in specific situations. Appropriately conveying this significant alliance is usually enough to settle team versus individual issues that may arise.

In addition, there is an underlying concern that needs to be factored into any decision—the consideration of short-term gain when returning to sport early versus long-term risks. Some long-term risks may have a lasting impact on an athlete's professional career. Some injuries can provoke issues that can be regarded as premature or career ending. For example, the development of degenerative joint disease and osteoarthritis-based problems could result at an earlier stage than normal. Evidence shows that such conditions can increase the risk of long-term disabilities and need to be considered by clinicians because of their immense impact both to the athlete and health care system. The sports therapist's clinical reasoning process must always take into consideration the short-term gain of returning to sport, and perhaps the glory that comes with it versus the potential global long-term adverse effects.

Preparation can improve clinical decision making

Improvements in the effectiveness of current injury treatments and their associated rehabilitation programs have increased resulting in an expectation of the return of injured athletes to sport within accelerated time frames. To match this shift in the athlete's condensed time out of sport, one has to improve one's awareness of overall injury and healing potential, as well as improve our knowledge of injury prevention and, in particular, an athlete's risk of reinjury.

During past Olympic Games, it has been a requirement of the Australian Olympic medical team to make a conscious effort to seek adequate medical and injury information on all Australian athletes or squads/teams under its care. It cannot be emphasized enough how important it is in preparation for any injury or illness scenarios that could arise during the Olympic Games period. For those involved as the principle sports medicine providers, this information can be essential to be able to appropriately address the question of when the athlete can return to sport.

It should come as no surprise that an athlete's previous injury history increases his or her risk of reinjury. Knowledge that is gained through the process of an athlete's precompetition medical or musculoskeletal screening could potentially minimize injury risks or, in the least, improve one's clinical decision making when dealing with potential ongoing injury sequences. If one of the medical aims at the Olympic Games is to be able to appropriately address the issue of an injured athlete's return to sport, having an adequate knowledge of past injuries, appropriate past treatments for specific conditions seem important.

An element of preinjury data is essential in the environment of elite sports competition. This is particularly evident in the bonding of various athletes from a wide scope of sports that converge during Olympic competition, especially due to the potentially fierce and unforgiving nature of the competition within a relatively short period.

Impact of the short time available to work within injury constraints and rehabilitation processes at an Olympic Game

One of the greatest challenges in a competition environment is to successfully return the athlete to competition following injury or keep the athlete competing with an injury. The clinician's clinical reasoning skills as well his/her ability to effectively use an assortment of treatment skills are often brought to test. It is important that the initial injury diagnosis is correct; this allows a more effective return to play consideration through the efficiency of an appropriate treatment plan. The pressures of major competition accentuate the need to work efficiently for short periods. These strict deadlines put pressure on the sports therapist's time management skills. The sports therapist must take care to ensure that these uncommon external stimuli occurring over short periods during competition do not inevitably lead to rushed and often poor clinical judgments. The key factor in these types of situations is not to let the circumstances overpower one's normal treatment processes and standards. High-level clinical judgment and reasoning skills must be used to enable the clinician to work more effectively. Many short-term, high-pressure rehabilitation periods require a greater array of treatment techniques that any single sports therapist may not possess. One should not be afraid to seek help and additional advice to successfully address the athlete's overall treatment plan and make use of the skill and techniques needed from a large selection of practitioners usually available at the games.

Normal injury management should continue even when working within shorter timelines. These include the need for adequate acute injury management and return of preinjury elements such as strength, flexibility, and proprioception following injury. Functional movements that are requirements of the athlete's sports also need to be restored. Not all tests give a clear outcome of performance levels, so if one is still in doubt, it is wise to lean toward safety rather than risk. The therapist again needs to balance these risks with those environmental and situational complexities that conflict with the decision to return an athlete to sport. It is also more effective if the medical team can observe recovering athletes within the field of training, similar to the environment they will be returning to; this allows for better understanding of their preparedness to return to sport.

Unfortunately, the pressures of the on-field decisions are even harder to master and their large scope of possibilities immediately evokes a new set of parameters. One must utilize the basic line of care in these situations, ensuring that the athlete's best interest and ultimate safety is the primary goal (Figure 9.6).

Communication of decisions with athlete, coach, team officials

Good, honest communication can help solve a number of issues before they gain momentum and interrupt appropriate athlete management decisions. First, one must work to gain the respect and alliance with the appropriate stakeholders, which should begin leading up to the event or in the early stages of competition. For most sports therapists working within the Olympic environment, this level of communication and respect should have already been attained due to their nomination and attendance as a team representative.

Second, all personnel dealing with athletic care should be involved in the process of gathering information on the athlete and his or her care. This may require one to engage outside specialists as required (e.g., sports psychology) to assist with outcome feedback and achieve the best care possible. The athlete should be involved in the decision-making process as well, as this can be an effective way of helping them to understand and accept the eventual outcome; this, however, may take good influencing skills. Communication is the key; therefore, to be effective, information should be conveyed to all parties in a manner that is easily understood and succinct.

In most cases, once the appropriate decision has been acknowledged and a transparent process has

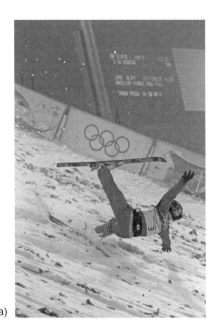

(a)

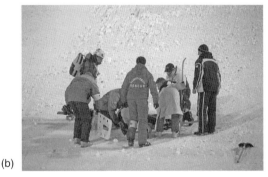

(b)

Figure 9.6 After a fall and injury (a), on-field emergency management of an injury (b), decision making regarding the injury, and determination of the athletes' ability to continue to compete are critical decisions that all sports medicine and sports therapy personnel must be able to make quickly and efficiently (Photos courtesy of the International Olympic Committee)

been shown for the benefit of all parties, a healthier situation is created especially if everyone is properly informed. If one is confident in the way one communicates, then there is a greater likelihood that the athlete will be confident in the decisions that are made.

Conflict of interest

At times, the decision-making process can become clouded or obstructed by the beliefs or expectations of one or various parties that may be involved. Careful delivery of return to sport decisions is required in sensitive or borderline situations. Athletes at every level of sport will always have fears of being taken out of competition.

> Doctors and scientists said that breaking the four minute mile was impossible. That one would die in the attempt. Thus when I got up from the track after collapsing at the finish line, I figured I was dead.
>
> Roger Banister
> Track and Field
> http://quotations.about.com/cs/
> inspirationquotes/a/Sports13.htm

Ethical dilemmas will arise when the decision of one person contradicts another's opinion on an issue. When dealing with athlete injuries, a key component is for the clinician to always show empathy and not sympathy with the athlete's plight. The clinician should always demonstrate exceptional communication skills throughout the process to limit the appearance of indecisiveness and to decrease the chances of misunderstanding. The clinician must show that he or she has analyzed the consequences of his/her decision from a professional standpoint and always considering what is best for an athlete from a health and safety point of view. By using this type of strategy, one can be confident that a sound decision has been made.

Where possible, the clinician should encourage the athlete, coach, or parent to limit "Doctor shopping" in which the athlete talks to several clinicians and takes the advice of the one who agrees most readily with what the athlete wants. This scenario will only cause issues and confusion as the athlete is still just seeking an answer that he or she wants to hear. In these instances, the clinician should approach the situation by offering to arrange for the athlete to meet with another practitioner to obtain another opinion, so that the athlete is assured that

all efforts are being made to make the right decision. The clinician should seek this help when he or she feels that there may be conflicting issues. In some cases, an appropriate outside opinion will give perspective to both parties.

If the therapist follows the ethical code of sports medicine by always making sure that the athlete's health is a priority and that one should do no harm, one can be confident that any decision is ethically correct.

Press and media scrutiny

The Olympic environment is one that generates a high level of media interest (see Figure 7.4). The lure of an Olympic gold and recognition of athletes' Olympic sporting achievement attracts worldwide attention. This interest can be both positive and negative depending on the situation. In many cases, an athlete's injury or withdrawal from competition can gain interest just short of what one could similarly achieve in Olympic glory. As a sports medicine practitioner, one needs to be aware of the possibility of drawing questions from the media.

The fundamental rule to follow when dealing with the media is to always have permission from both the athlete and team management before discussing any injury situations with the media. One should remember that, in most cases, it is much safer to decline to talk to media about specific cases and leave all the communications in the hands of the team's media staff.

Key concerns of the sports therapist at major events/competitions

The Olympic Games are always going to create greater pressures on all involved including the therapists and medical team through the perceived stakes of competition and expectations of others to perform and succeed. Return to play decisions may also have a major impact on an Olympic-based athlete's possible income, endorsements, and career benefits. Getting any decision correct is vital for the long-term prospects of the athlete as well as the short-term glory.

Consistent peak competitive performance loads over extended periods can contribute to high injury rates in an elite sports population. Similarly, the Olympic competition can be the accumulation of long periods of other competitions, training, and preparation. The role of the sports physiotherapist is to give the injured athlete every chance to compete, but there are certain limitations as to how much can be achieved, even at such times as an Olympic final.

In the end, the same professional approach is being asked of clinicians, but with the Olympics and other major competitions, there is a higher focus within an environment of elevated intensity. The clinician must evaluate the situation and attenuate to those unusual aspects that create good clinical reasoning skills when dealing with treatment and an athlete's return to competition or training. The clinician must work effectively and in a succinct fashion with meaningful purpose.

The most important thing in the Olympic Games is not to win, but to take part, just as the most important thing in life is not to triumph, but the struggle. The essential thing is not to have conquered, but to have fought well (Figure 9.7).

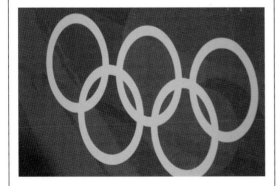

Figure 9.7 Olympic rings

Baron Pierre de Coubertin
Founder of the modern Olympic movement
http://quotations.about.com/od/
sportsquotes/a/olympics2.htm

The athletes' follow-up

An athlete's return to activity or sport does not end the responsibility of the medical staff. In fact, it can have the opposite effect where it requires a heightened attentiveness to the athlete's situation. Follow-up is an important aspect in the ongoing management of the athlete and should never be overlooked even after the athlete's event or competition phase has ended. Reports and handover information are seen at times as a task but is essential in transparent treatment of athlete injuries.

Rehabilitation and maintenance treatment are required to continue the athlete's return to sport. In many cases, when an athlete returns to competition or practice, there are ongoing issues, including the potential risk of reinjury or a new injury. Clinicians have a responsibility to ensure an athlete's ongoing treatment or rehabilitation requirements are successful in maintaining them in continued activity. When one is working within the elite athlete environment, stricter guidelines in the form of postinjury rehabilitation protocols should be the standard outline followed after injury to ensure effectiveness. From the information presented within this chapter, one should ascertain that the process of making a decision on an athlete's return to sport is not an exact science. Instead it relies on expert opinion as well as using a thoughtful and highly informed process of clinical reasoning and evaluation. Essentially, each case of returning to sport must be assessed within its own merits, highlighting the aspects that emphasize the specific situations and environment. There is no recipe or outline that can be given that could solve every return to sport scenario.

However, establishing a transparent process of decision making early within a team or sporting event is essential for its overall effectiveness when a decision needs to be made about returning an athlete to sport.

In the end, a decision must essentially revolve around ensuring the best interest of the athlete as the primary goal, which ultimately is the safety of the athlete. With this basic reasoning, the outcome of a game, winning or losing, should never be an issue in a return to compete scenario. By conveying the ultimate outcome in a clear and confident way, the process will seem straightforward.

References

Brukner, P. & Khan, K. (2007) *Clinical Sports Medicine*, 3rd Edn. McGraw-Hill, Australia.

Creighton, D.W., Shrier, I., Shultz, R., Meeuwisse, W.H. & Matheson, G.O. (2010) Return to play: a decision based model. *Clinical Sports Medicine*, 20, 379–385.

Herring, S., Bergfeld, J., Boyd, J., Duffey, T., Fields, K.B., Grana, W.A., Indelicato, P., Kibler, W.B., Pallay, R., Putukian, M. & Sallis, R.E. (2002) The team physician and return-to-play issues: a consensus statement. *Medicine and Science in Sports and Exercise*, 34, 1212–1214.

Higgs, J., Jones, M.A., Loftus, S. & Christensen, N. (2008) *Clinical Reasoning in Health Professionals*, 3rd Edn. Elsevier Health Sciences, Australia.

Verrall, G.M., Kalairajah, Y., Slavotinek, J.P. & Spriggins, A.J. (2006) Assessment of player performance following return to sport after hamstring muscle strain injury. *Journal of Science and Medicine in Sport*, 9, 87–90.

Chapter 10
Sports nutrition and therapy

Louise Burke[1] and Ron Maughan[2]

[1] Australian Sports Commission, Bruce, ACT, Australia
[2] Loughborough University, Loughborough, UK

Introduction

Although athletes are now aware of the importance of nutrition in supporting training and promoting optimal performance during competition, its role in the management of the times when the athlete is unable to train or compete is less well appreciated. Nevertheless, there are a number of ways in which careful attention to eating and, perhaps, judicious use of supplements can assist in the recovery from injury and in the reduction of risk of future injuries. The aim of this review is to cover the nutritional needs of "rehab" (repair/regeneration from injury) and "prehab" (preventing future injury or reducing atrophy following scheduled surgery). In addition, it will address the challenges of managing energy balance during periods of reduced energy expenditure, including the temptation to "comfort eat" while adjusting to the emotional toll of sporting injuries.

Repair and regeneration of injured tissues

Sports injuries can both result from, or cause, suboptimal form and function of body tissues. Although acute or chronic trauma to bone, muscle, tendon, or other soft tissue is most often identi-fied as the cause of interruption to an athlete's training or competition, it is better seen as part of a "vicious cycle" of problems. Injury is associated with removal or reduction of an accustomed training stimulus, leading to significant atrophy in the architecture and function of body tissues. Immobilization due to bed rest or limb rest/casting represents an extreme withdrawal of this stimulus and causes rapid impairments to muscle, tendon, and bone. The loss of function associated with injury relates not only to strength, power, or ability to perform exercise activities but also to the loss of muscle oxidative capacity and metabolic flexibility.

The repair of an acute injury is usually divided into two phases. The first or immediate phase encompasses tissue repair, immobilization, and atrophy. Tissue repair itself involves overlapping processes of inflammation (defense against microorganisms and initiation of healing), proliferation (e.g., initiation of scar tissue, synthesis of protein and collagen, deposition of calcium in bone), and remodeling periods (finalization and maturation of new tissues). The atrophy or tissue wasting that occurs during this first phase is affected by the loss of activity/loading, and nutritional goals include the minimization of loss of protein and bone demineralization. The second phase in injury repair is the rehabilitation or "rehab" of the affected parts as the athlete prioritizes the loading on tissues and tries to reverse the loss of form and function. This phase also involves a net increase in

Sports Therapy Services, First Edition. Edited by James E. Zachazewski and David J. Magee.
© 2012 International Olympic Committee. Published 2012 by John Wiley & Sons, Ltd.

protein-containing tissues such as bone, tendon, and muscle, with other goals being to promote mineralization of bone. Finally, many athletes also undertake proactive programs ("prehab") to promote muscle and bone strength in order to resist injury or in the case of scheduled surgery, to try to limit the anticipated degree of postoperative atrophy

Nutritional strategies to protect muscle protein balance

The atrophy of tissue mass and function during injury and immobilization results from an alteration in the balance between protein synthesis and breakdown. Although many people assume that muscle wasting is due to an acceleration of protein breakdown, recent studies have provided consistent evidence that it is principally caused by a decline in the synthesis of new muscle proteins both in fasting and fed states. In fact, in humans, there is generally a *reduction* in protein breakdown during injury, but since this is less than the reduction in synthesis, the net result is negative protein balance. Countermeasures should, therefore, target strategies to enhance muscle protein synthesis rather than those that attempt to counteract protein breakdown. In other words, injury repair and minimization of muscle wasting is best undertaken using the same strategies that underpin the process of training: the combination of muscle overload via resistance training and nutrient support. While physical therapists and strength and conditioning coaches will need to design an appropriate exercise program for the injured athlete, nutritional strategies around this program will play a role in the effectiveness of the outcomes.

Protein and Essential Amino Acids. It is readily apparent that regular exercise has a number of highly specific effects on body protein turnover. Strength training, for example, results in increases in muscle mass, indicating an increased formation of actin and myosin, while endurance training increases the muscle content of mitochondrial proteins, especially those involved in oxidative metabolism. Collagen is the connective tissue protein that is important for tendons and ligaments. Enhanced recovery and repair from injury requires an enhancement of protein synthesis both to reduce the initial loss of tissue protein and to rebuild new tissues during the rehabilitation phase.

Although the historical interest in protein needs for sport became largely stalled by debates on total protein intake/requirements over the day, more recent investigations of acute protein intake around an exercise session have produced strategies which promote clear benefits to the outcomes of a single workout and chronic training programs. Sophisticated studies have shown that protein synthesis and breakdown are elevated after a bout of resistance exercise, with catabolism dominating in the fasted state. However, the intake of protein, or more specifically, the intake of essential amino acids including leucine, promotes protein synthesis leading to a net muscle protein gain. Studies show that benefits are optimized with the intake of as little as 20–25 g of high-quality protein (equivalent to approximately 6–8 g of essential amino acids) soon after exercise. Furthermore, recovery meals/snacks based on dairy protein and, in particular, the fast-digesting whey protein component, provide an effective dietary choice to optimize protein synthesis after exercise. Indeed, studies in previously sedentary people have shown that the combination of resistance exercise and a dairy/whey protein recovery drink achieves greater gains in lean body mass and a reduction in body fat than an isocaloric treatment featuring a carbohydrate drink with soy protein/milk achieving intermediate results. Table 10.1 provides examples of meal/snacks providing 20 g of high-quality protein.

The elevation in protein synthesis following an acute bout of exercise is known to continue for up to 24 hours following this stimulus, meaning that future guidelines for optimal protein intakes for athletes might include recommendations for the timing and quantity of protein intake over the whole of the day. Although definite guidelines are still premature, it seems prudent to combine a protein-rich recovery snack with a meal pattern that spreads protein intake more evenly over the day than is currently observed in most Western cultures. It is also likely that athletes meet their protein needs over a wide range of total daily protein intakes, with intakes of 1.2–2 g/kg or approximately 200% of population guidelines for protein

Table 10.1 Examples of dietary choices providing 20 g of high-quality program

Food	Amount Needed to Provide 20-g Protein
Single foods (note that food composition may vary between products from different countries)	• 3 medium eggs • 500–600 mL reduced or low-fat milk • 60 g (3 slices) of reduced fat cheese • 140-g cottage cheese • 400–500 g low-fat fruit yogurt • 500-mL low-fat custard • 70-g lean beef, lamb, or pork (cooked weight) • 80-g lean chicken (cooked weight) • 100-g grilled fish • 100–180 g canned tuna or salmon (drained weight) • 50-g skim milk powder
Supplements/sports foods (note that these are an expensive alternative to food)	• 30–40 g high protein powder or protein hydrolysate • 250–300 mL liquid meal supplement • 20–30 g high protein sports bar
Examples of food combinations and less expensive alternatives to supplements	• Meat and cheese sandwich (moderate thickness filling of 20-g cheese slices + 50 g filling) • Small bowl of cereal with 200-g carton of yogurt + skim milk hot chocolate • Cheese omelet (2 large eggs + 20-g cheese) • 100-g tin tuna on crackers + 200 mL glass milk • 500-mL homemade fruit smoothie (recipe: 250-mL low-fat milk, 200-g fruit yogurt, 1 banana or cup berries) • 400-mL fortified milk shake (= 300-mL low-fat flavored milk + 2 tablespoons ice cream + 25-g skim milk powder)

being typical of the otherwise well-chosen dietary practices of athletes across a range of sports.

Since protein is only stored in tissues in a functional role, higher protein diets are associated with upregulation of enzymes responsible for protein oxidation to allow high rates of disposal of the excess amino acids. This may not be a problem if high protein intakes are consumed chronically. However, a sudden drop in habitual protein intake would be expected to exacerbate the loss of muscle mass caused by the cessation or reduction in training stimulus. This is an important consideration, since many injured athletes dramatically alter their eating habits or supplement use when training is suspended. It seems prudent if athletes need to reduce their energy intake, either to promote weight loss or to maintain energy balance during a period of reduced energy expenditure; the level of protein intake should be maintained while energy intakes are adjusted by a reduced intake of other macronutrients. Indeed, studies of weight loss in athletes show that there appears to be some value in maintaining

daily protein intakes at the upper end of the range of 1.2–2 g/kg to preserve muscle mass. This might also apply to periods of preserving protein status during injury.

There is some debate regarding the value of special protein supplements to assist in the achievement of protein needs of athletes. In general, a range of wholesome foods can provide protein intake targets at the same time as supplying a source of other important nutrients. The advantages of "real foods" included cost-effectiveness, the achievement of multiple nutritional goals, and the benefits of social eating and food enjoyment. On the other hand, simple sports supplements such as whey protein powders offer the convenience of simple storage and preparation requirements and a known nutrient dose, which may justify their additional expense in certain situations. The least justifiable products are expensive supplements containing a range of other compounds that claim to enhance muscle protein synthesis or reduce breakdown. As will be discussed later, evidence to support the claims made for the majority of these products is weak or absent. One exception to this rule might be amino acid supplements providing leucine or essential amino acids to meet the dose outlined earlier. This could be of use in situations where the athlete with reduced energy expenditure wants to meet the protein needs of optimal muscle support with the lowest cost. Nevertheless, the specific value of such supplements is yet to be determined and it is likely that expert advice from a sports dietitian will allow the athlete to develop eating patterns that integrate a large range of dietary goals more efficiently and cost-effectively.

Energy Intake. Energy intake is important during repair and rehabilitation of injury for a variety of reasons that will be covered in more detail later. Underpinning themes include the two different but interrelated concepts of energy availability and energy balance (Table 10.2). There are consequences to protein synthesis and balance if energy availability is threatened (i.e., energy intake is reduced below the level that is able to support the health and maintenance needs of the body) and/or the athlete is in energy deficit to lose weight. As discussed earlier, higher protein intakes of approximately 2 g/kg/d may help to preserve protein status in athletes undertaking a period of energy deficit; however, mild energy deficit and resistance exercise are necessary factors to minimize net loss of muscle protein. An injured or immobile athlete who has a limited ability to undertake appropriate exercise will already be subject to protein loss and, for many reasons that are covered in this review, should not further exacerbate protein wasting by deliberately undertaking weight loss during this period.

Other Amino Acids. Arginine and ornithine are reported to stimulate growth hormone release and to promote growth of lean tissue when taken during a period of strength training. There is some published evidence to support this, but any increase in growth hormone secretion is small compared with that which results from a bout of high-intensity exercise. A number of other amino acids, including histidine, lysine, methionine, and phenylalanine, are sold as "anabolic agents," but there is little reason

to believe that specific supplementation with these amino acid will promote gains in muscle mass.

Micronutrients. There is good evidence that zinc is important in helping the tissue repair process that is an important part of recovery following traumatic injury. The processes of breakdown of damaged cells and tissues after injury and the manufacture of new tissues are in some ways similar to those that occur with training. Most of the remodeling involves changes to the proteins in tissue, but other cellular components are also involved. Studies on young children, where rapid tissue growth is ideally taking place, show that zinc deficiency results in a failure to grow normally, combined with loss of appetite and signs of poor wound healing.

The need for zinc supplements during rehabilitation from injury (or indeed training) is often based on the flawed assumption that excess intake can enhance muscle growth and repair. However, zinc supplementation is likely to be of benefit only when an inadequacy is present. Zinc is found in a range of sources in the diet, including meat, fish, seafood, legumes, and whole grain cereals. Nutritional assessment and counseling will allow the athlete to achieve an intake that is adequate in amount and availability. Where a preexisting deficiency has developed from a diet low in energy and/or variety, or is at risk because of inability to correct these dietary risk factors, a zinc supplement may be prescribed.

Deficiencies of a number of other micronutrients, including vitamins A and C, will also slow the healing process after damage to muscle. For example, vitamin C is important in the synthesis of collagen. Although micronutrient deficiencies are rare in healthy athletic populations, athletes are often encouraged to take megadoses of these nutrients to prevent injury or to promote repair. There is no evidence for any beneficial effects of large doses of any of these or any other single nutrients. Instead the preferred option is for athletes to consume a plentiful intake of vitamins, minerals, and other potentially helpful phytonutrients from a variety of food sources, with a prudent use of supplements to support low energy intakes and restricted dietary range where justified.

Table 10.2 Definitions of energy balance and energy availability

Definition	Principle	Calculation	Examples	Comments
Energy balance	Determines loss or gain of body tissue	Energy intake—total energy expenditure (energy cost of resting metabolic rate + exercise + cost of daily living activities + thermic effect of food + growth)	• Total energy expenditure including cost of exercise = 1500 kcal/d (6300 kJ) • Total energy intake = 2500 kcal/d (10,500 kJ) = negative energy balance (deficit) of 1000 kcal (4200 kJ) per day	Loss of body mass from body fat and muscle mass depending on exercise stimulus, degree and spread of energy deficit over the day, genetic variability, and other factors
			• Total energy expenditure including cost of exercise = 2500 kcal/d (10,500 kJ) • Total energy intake = 2500 kcal/d (10,500 kJ) = energy balance	Generally, there should be little change in body mass
			• Total energy expenditure including cost of exercise = 1500 kcal/d (6300 kJ) • Total energy intake = 3000 kcal/d (12,600) = positive energy balance (surplus) of 500 kcal (2100 kJ) per day	Gain in body mass from body fat and muscle mass depending on exercise stimulus, degree and spread of energy surplus over the day, genetic variability, and other factors
Energy availability	Determines how much energy the body can devote to everyday functions of health and maintenance	Energy intake = energy cost of daily exercise (expressed per kg of athlete's fat-free mass [FFM])		
		>45 kcal (189 kJ) per kg FFM		Weight gain, growth, hypertrophy
		~ 45 kcal (189 kJ) per kg FFM		Healthy, weight maintenance
		30–45 kcal (125–189 kJ) per kg FFM	Athlete A: 55 kg (20% body fat = 80% FFM); Weekly training = 5600 kcal (23.5 MJ); Daily energy intake = 2520 kcal (10.6 MJ) Energy availability = (2520–800)/(0.8 × 55) = 39 kcal/kg FFM (164 kJ)	Healthy weight loss (or weight maintenance at reduced metabolic rate)
		<30 kcal (125 kJ) per kg FFM	Athlete B: 55 kg (25% body fat = 75% FFM) Weekly training = 5600 kcal (2.35 MJ) Daily energy intake = 1980 kcal (8.3 MJ) Energy availability = (1980–800)/(0.75 × 55) = 29 kcal/kg FFM (120 kJ)	Low energy availability with potential consequences to bone health, metabolic rate, reproductive hormones and other body systems

Special Supplements for Enhanced Protein Balance. Creatine is one of a few nutritional ergogenic aids that is supported by a large body of credible evidence, justifying the popularity of its use by athletes, particularly in strength and power sports. Muscle creatine—in the form of phosphocreatine—is an important energy source for high-intensity exercise. The diet of meat eaters typically provides about half of the daily creatine requirement of about 2 g with the remainder being synthesized from amino acid precursors. Vegetarians typically have lower muscle creatine stores due to their reliance on this de novo synthesis. Supplementation for a few days with a high-dose creatine supplement (10–20 g/day in 2–4 divided doses) or for a longer period (about 30 days) with a smaller daily dose (3 g/day) can result in substantial increases (typically 10–30%) in the muscle creatine content. This promotes the regeneration of muscle phosphocreatine stores after high-intensity exercise, which in turn enhances the performance of repeated bouts of high-intensity exercise with short recovery intervals such as interval training, resistance training, and the game characteristics of intermittent team and racquet sports. Athletes who use creatine supplements typically gain body mass—usually in the order of 2–4 kg. There is still debate on the exact contribution to this gain from several sources including water retention in the muscle, the direct effect of creatine supplements on muscle protein synthesis, or enhanced support of resistance training. Therefore, creatine supplementation may enhance the results of rehabilitation programs undertaken to restore muscle size and mass following injury.

There have been few studies on the use of creatine supplementation to maintain or increase muscle mass and function during periods of disuse or to reduce the loss of muscle that occurs with injury or immobilization. Furthermore, the results of these studies are contradictory with some showing benefits while others fail to see differences with creatine treatment. In one study, Hespel *et al.* (2001) immobilized one leg of healthy volunteers for a period of 2 weeks, resulting in a loss of muscle cross-sectional area (CSA) of about 900 mm^2 and a loss of about 30 W in a test of knee extension power output. This was followed by a 10-week rehabilitation period in which subjects received either a placebo or a creatine supplement. Recovery of both muscle mass, as measured by CSA, and functional capacity as measured by peak power output was faster and more complete with the creatine supplement than with placebo. The same authors showed that creatine supplementation can offset the decline in muscle GLUT4 protein content that occurs during immobilization and can increase GLUT4 protein content during subsequent rehabilitation training in healthy subjects. It is less certain that the initial loss of muscle can be prevented by creatine supplementation, but these results do suggest a role during the rehabilitation phase after surgery or other injury.

β-Hydroxy, β-methylbutyrate (HMB) is a metabolite of the amino acid leucine and is sold as a promoter of muscle growth via a reduction in protein catabolism. There are also claims that it can reduce body fat, stimulate the immune system, and produce beneficial effects on the coronary risk profile of the blood lipids. The evidence is not entirely convincing, but there is some support for a positive effect on muscle mass in conjunction with the onset of a training program. Whether this evidence is strong enough to warrant the use of HMB for injury rehabilitation remains uncertain.

Some recent evidence suggests that a few weeks of supplementation with omega-3 fatty acids from fish oils can stimulate muscle protein synthesis via an enhancement of muscle signaling pathways. This has been confirmed in more than one study, but as with so much else in this field, this supplementation has not been investigated in elite athletes undergoing intensive training or in individuals after injury or after surgery.

Nutrients with anti-inflammatory properties

Some food components can be shown to have antioxidant or anti-inflammatory actions when studied in isolated cell or tissue preparation agents; these include polyphenols such as green tea extract or curcumin and omega-3 fatty acids. Such results are often used in promoting the sale of these products. It has to be recognized, however, that there are many obstacles to the application of these findings to the intact human. The bioavailability of many preparations is low and there may be no perceptible change in blood or tissue concentrations after ingestion. In some cases, the concentration shown to be effective in vitro is many times higher than the maximum concentration that can be achieved in vivo.

It has to be recognized as well that the inflammatory process is an essential part of tissue repair and that free radicals and other reactive oxygen species are generated by cells of the immune system as part of their defense against invading pathogens. Blocking these actions by the use of high doses of antioxidants and anti-inflammatory agents may therefore alleviate some of the symptoms but may actually be counterproductive. This uncertainty presents a dilemma for the athlete and for those who advise them. It seems sensible to choose foods that are high in antioxidants and anti-inflammatories, such as whole grains, fruits, vegetables, nuts, and seeds, but it is less certain that supplements will be beneficial. High doses of single antioxidants may do more harm than good.

Bone and connective tissue

During periods of immobilization or inactivity, the mechanical stress on bone is removed and some loss of bone mass is likely to occur. Where mechanical loading of the bone is not an option, nutritional strategies to maintain the health of bone and connective tissue become particularly important. A wide range of dietary factors will influence the health and function of these tissues, including energy intake, and the intakes of protein, calcium, zinc, magnesium, and vitamins A, B, and K. There is also some evidence that a high intake of fruits and vegetables may benefit bone health, either by the effects of acid–base status or because of their phytoestrogen content.

Energy Availability and Protein. Energy intake plays an important role in bone health with even mild reductions in energy availability having a direct role in increasing bone turnover, principally by reducing bone formation. Although measurable effects become apparent only after relatively long periods of time, even short periods of severe energy restriction, as may happen in the injured athlete seeking to limit the gain of body fat, may have adverse effects on bone health. It is well established that an adequate dietary protein intake is essential for good bone health. Insufficient protein intake is detrimental to the acquisition of bone mass during periods of rapid bone growth in childhood and adolescence. Low dietary protein intakes are also associated with a failure to preserve bone mass in older adults.

Calcium and Vitamin D. Adequate intakes of vitamin D and calcium are essential for bone health, but high intakes do not necessarily indicate adequate status. Vitamin D is essential for maintaining normal calcium metabolism and a major purpose of vitamin D is to increase intestinal calcium absorption. Only about 10–15% of the calcium from the diet is absorbed in individuals who are deficient in vitamin D, while 30–35% is absorbed when vitamin D status is adequate. Low calcium intakes and poor vitamin D status may result in a loss of bone mass and an increased risk for stress fractures. Vitamin D is also now known to play a number of important roles in areas other than bone health, including a role in the regulation of anti-inflammatory responses and immune function and in skeletal muscle growth.

There is growing evidence that vitamin D insufficiency may be widespread among athletes as well as in the general population. Dietary sources of vitamin D are limited, fatty fish and egg yolk being the only common sources in the diet, but fortification of foods in some countries can supply greater amounts. Nevertheless, direct exposure to the UVB radiation from sunshine is the principle source of vitamin D for most people. Athletes at risk of vitamin D insufficiency or deficiency include those who train indoors or with strict attention to skin cancer prevention strategies, those who live at high latitudes where sunshine exposure is low for large parts of the year and those with dark skin pigmentation. Poor vitamin D status might increase the risk of injury if it impairs bone and muscle health; however, injury might also increase the risk of vitamin D status if immobilization or altered lifestyle reduces sunshine exposure. Measurement of vitamin D status in athletes at risk may help to identify those who need supplementation as part of an injury prevention strategy or as therapy during recovery from injury. Poor vitamin D status has also been associated with an increased frequency of illness in collegiate athletes.

Supplements for Bone and Joint Health. A wide range of dietary supplements is sold with claims that they can enhance or maintain bone and joint health. An extensive range of such things as herbs and botanicals are also sold including turmeric, Boswellia serrata, Cayenne pepper, Ashwagandha, autumn crocus, meadowsweet, stinging nettle, willow bark (Salix), and devil's claw. Animal extracts, including green-lipped mussel and sea cucumber, are also promoted. The most popular supplement, however, is glucosamine that is often sold in combination with chondroitin.

The cartilage in joints is made up of proteoglycans and the protein collagen. Proteoglycans consist of a protein molecule bound to various complex sugars known as glycosaminoglycans. Chondroitin is a common glycosaminoglycan, with commercial preparations being extracted from the cartilaginous tissues of animals. Glucosamine is a carbohydrate–amino compound that is produced from the chitin that forms the main structural element of seashells. Both compounds are reported to stimulate the formation of components of cartilage when given orally to humans. There is now a considerable amount of information from clinical trials involving patients with osteoarthritis to show that regular (once or twice per day) long-term (about 2–6 months) treatment with glucosamine and chondroitin sulfate can reduce the severity of subjective symptoms. There is no evidence at present of a benefit for athletes with joint pain, but there seem to have been no properly controlled trials in athletes. One study of US military special operations personnel with knee and back pain showed subjective improvements after treatment but no effect on tests of running performance.

A large-scale trial on the use of glucosamine–chondroitin supplementation (the GAIT study (Glucosamine/Chondroitin Arthritis Intervention Trial)) showed that overall there were no significant differences between the placebo and supplemented groups. For a subset of participants with moderate-to-severe pain, glucosamine combined with chondroitin sulfate provided statistically significant pain relief compared with placebo (about 79% had a 20% or greater reduction in pain versus about 54% for placebo). For participants in the mild pain subset, glucosamine and chondroitin sulfate together or alone did not provide statistically significant pain relief. There may be some individuals who experience subjective relief from the use of glucosamine, and it seems to do no harm.

There has been much recent interest in the role of various phytochemicals in reducing the inflammatory responses that accompany injury to tendons as well as to muscle. As mentioned earlier, however, many compounds can be shown to have anti-inflammatory properties, and some show promising results in laboratory models, but few have been investigated for their potential in randomized control studies. For example, curcumin, which is responsible for the bright yellow color of the spice turmeric, has recently been shown to inhibit inflammation and cell death induced by inflammatory agents in tendons grown in tissue culture. It remains to be seen, though, whether this will have measurable beneficial effects in injured tendons. Included in the discussion should be the issue of whether inhibition of inflammation is always a positive strategy since it is part of the process of injury repair. It is possible that compounds that dampen this aspect of the process may, in fact, interfere with some of its positive roles.

Adjusting energy and nutrient intake to altering requirements

A noticeable feature of periods of injury and rehabilitation is the alteration, often dramatic, of an athlete's exercise program, and thus energy expenditure. According to the seriousness of the problem and the phase of its management, the injured athlete can expect to experience significant changes to both the energy cost of exercise (both sporting and rehabilitation programs) and their activities of daily living. Table 10.3 summarizes the common ways

Table 10.3 Common situations of changing components in energy balance related to injury

Issue	Change from Habitual Patterns	Comments	Suggestions
Energy expenditure			
Cessation or modification to the normal training and competition program	Decrease		The athlete needs to be aware of this decrease in energy expenditure and should try to adjust energy intake toward this change
Addition of rehabilitation program of resistance or conditioning exercise	Decrease or increase	May be less than habitual exercise but increased initial level above. In some cases, may be higher than habitual level if added to normal training as "prehab" or undertaken by athlete whose habitual training is skill based	See above. Note that it will be important to adjust for the increased cost of rehabilitation training to ensure optimal adaptation
Energy cost of wound/injury repair	Increase	Many of biochemical and physiological processes of healing are highly energy costing	It is important not to be in a situation of low-energy availability or energy deficit so that repair processes are suboptimal
Interference with normal activities of daily living due to reduced mobility/immobility or due to busy timetable associated with injury management	Decrease		The athlete needs to be aware of this decrease in energy expenditure and should try to adjust energy intake or undertake alternative appropriate activities
Energy cost of using wheelchair or crutches	Increase	This energy cost is often forgotten	
Energy intake			
Comfort eating: unusual or increased intake of energy dense foods and alcohol	Increase	Often associated with psychological release from the rigors of sporting commitment or as a coping mechanism for frustration and disappointment	The athlete needs to find alternative options to cope with the emotional side of injury. Counseling may be valuable. It is also possible to find "comfort foods" that are compatible with new nutritional goals
Social eating: increased opportunity for food intake as entertainment.	Increase	Often due to lack of structure in day or need to find new activities to fill in the time usually committed to sport	The athlete needs to find alternative options to cope with time management and entertainment. Counseling may be valuable. It is also possible to find social eating options that are compatible with new nutritional goals

(Continued)

Table 10.3 *(Continued)*

Issue	Change from Habitual Patterns	Comments	Suggestions
Loss of appetite	Decrease	Often associated with reduced activity levels, pain, or side effects of medication	Menu planning should include foods that are easy to consume including well-liked and flavorsome options
Loss of intake associated with the usual habits of eating pre-, during, and postexercise	Decrease	Many athletes consume food/drinks to provide nutritional support for training sessions and competitions. Although this is generally a suitable way to track energy intake with energy needs, in some cases, eating around exercise contributes heavily to residual energy and nutrient needs and needs to be replaced with other eating opportunities	It is generally valuable for an athlete to attach eating occasions to exercise sessions. Apart from providing specific nutritional support for the session, this principle allows energy and nutrient intake to increase to match additional costs/requirements due to exercise. In some situations associated with injury, however, such a plan may need to be revised
Interference with access to food or appropriate food due to interference with domestic routines	Decrease	The athlete may have physical limitations to their ability to shop or cook for themselves while injured. They may also have an increase in their schedule due to the commitment to injury management that may interfere with preparing or eating meals/snacks	The athlete may need support to reorganize their access to food, or assistance with time management to allow all commitments to be met in the new daily timetable
Deliberate (over)restriction of energy intake to prevent gain of body fat (or even lose body fat) during injury	Decrease	Many athletes misunderstand their new energy requirements or fail to appreciate that restrictive eating can compromise injury repair and rehabilitation goals. Some are motivated by an irrational fear of fat gain, and others may consider a period out of sporting competition to be a challenge to "fix up" their perceived failings	Expert advice may help the athlete to negotiate an eating plan that prioritizes their real goals for recovery from injury and allows them to choose a more appropriate time and method to address physique goals

in which energy expenditure/requirements can either increase or decrease compared with habitual patterns due to features of an injury and its management. At the same time, there are also factors that consciously or unconsciously change in relation to eating patterns that can also change energy intake in either direction. The size and continu-ally altering nature of these changes, and the focus on the injury rather than other aspects of the athlete's life, can often mean that the athlete's diet becomes inappropriate in energy and nutrient content. This has consequences to the management of the present injury, the risk of future injuries, and the athlete's ability to meet nutrition goals related to his or her sport, particularly the maintenance of optimal physique.

Injury is usually a time of alteration in an athlete's physique with the degree of change being influenced by size and duration of alterations to the athlete's diet and exercise program. The immobilization and detraining aspects of the injury are typically associated with loss of muscle size and mass, while the energy imbalance usually favors gain of body fat. In some cases, these changes can be rapid and dramatic. In other cases, these changes may be largely unnoticed by the athlete since they may not lead to major net changes in body mass (i.e., the loss of muscle mass is roughly equivalent to the gain in body fat). Since lean mass and body fat are often important in the performance of a sport, this is an unwelcome change for the athlete. In fact, physique alterations resulting from a period of injury may contribute to the difficulties many athletes face in attempting to return to their previous levels of competition. Loss of muscle mass and strength/power can reduce performance, as can the loss of mobility or speed resulting from a gain in body fat. Both of these can increase the likelihood of further injury, either directly or indirectly, as a result of further loss of tissue protein and mineralization from the excessive overtraining or undereating that is undertaken to try to quickly alter physique.

The injured athlete must find a balanced approach to promoting a nutritional environment that promotes repair and regeneration, minimizes the wasting associated with a reduced training stimulus, and yet minimizes unnecessary gain of body fat. Certainly, it is appropriate for the athletes to adjust an energy intake needed to support a high exercise load, to an intake that is more commensurate with their new energy needs. However, it is important that neither energy intake nor nutrient support is restricted too heavily during the early recovery phase. As outlined earlier, adequate intake of energy and protein is important to support optimal rates of repair and regeneration. Although some athletes abandon any concern about energy balance, a more prudent approach may be to attempt to remain in energy balance during this phase or allow a small energy surplus to ensure adequate intakes of protein and other nutrients. In cases where restrained eating and low-energy availability have preceded

the injury and, probably contributed to it, expert assessment and counseling will be required to adjust energy and nutrient intakes toward a healthier long-term approach. It should be appreciated that athletes may be in states of low energy availability without being in energy deficit; this occurs if restrained eating practices have led to a reduction in metabolic rate so that energy intake now balances energy expenditure, but is too low to sustain optimal health and body function (see Table 10.2). Later phases of the rehabilitation may be more appropriate times to attempt correction of suboptimal physique issues along with general and then more specific conditioning.

A sports dietitian or nutrition expert will be able to assist the athlete to develop a nutrition plan that can evolve with the changing goals of injury repair and rehabilitation. This plan will be specific to each individual athlete and must balance the issues involved with appropriate energy intake, adequate intake of protein and other nutrients, altered ability to prepare food, considerations related to the psychology of eating, and time management needs. Issues that will need to be addressed are included in the considerations outlined in Table 10.3.

Communication between nutritionist/dietician and sports therapy team

This review has identified a large range of issues involved in the optimization of nutrition to prevent and treat injuries in athletes. A compelling case has been made for implementation of eating practices that will promote good health, injury resistance, sound training, and speedy recovery between workouts. Although the development of a flexible and adapting eating plan and its monitoring will benefit from the expertise of a sports dietitian, a variety of professionals should be involved in a multidisciplinary approach to implementing the plan and supporting the athlete's ability to achieve it. To conclude this review, we provide a summary of the roles that should be played within this team in Table 10.4.

Table 10.4 Roles played by multidisciplinary team members in promoting nutrition for injury prevention/treatment

Professional	Expertise or Opportunities in Sports Nutrition	Roles in Promoting Nutrition in Injury Prevention/Treatment
Sport nutritionist or dietitian (abbreviated to sports dietitian)	• Has specialist qualifications or expertise in – assessment of nutrient needs and nutrient status, – dietary survey methodology, – diet therapy in disease, – counseling, – food composition, – food and supplement standards, or – food preparation and handling	• Undertakes nutrition screening or dietary survey of team • Provides nutritional assessment and counseling of individual athletes • Develops nutrition policies for team or sporting group (e.g., body composition guidelines, supplement use) • Develops nutrition education resources and activities • Educates other members of sports medicine or sport science network regarding best practice in sports nutrition • Cooperates with medical team to plan and implement nutrition program to optimize injury management for individual athletes
Sports physician	• Often is the primary appointment of a sporting team or first point contact for an athlete seeking help for problem • Often is appointed as head of multidisciplinary sports medicine or sport science support team for athletic group or team or case management of individual athlete • Often travels with team or is sited at field of play during team training/competition, thus seeing nutrition practice firsthand • Is able to approve a variety of relevant diagnostic tests (e.g., hematology, biochemistry, bone density tests) • May not have studied nutrition or sports nutrition in depth	• Identifies need for specialized nutrition activities leading to referral to sports dietitian • Organizes appropriate diagnostic tests to allow or confirm diagnosis of nutrition-related medical problems (e.g., vitamin D deficiency, poor bone status, menstrual dysfunction) • Provides case management of individuals with complex medical problems (e.g., female athlete triad), as head of multidisciplinary team providing holistic approach to treatment • Where in close access to athletes in daily training environment or travel, implements or monitors team nutrition plan—often acting as the "eyes" or "hands" of the team sports dietitian who has organized plan
Sport physiotherapist or physical therapist	• Often provides lengthy individual treatments that provide rapport between athlete and therapist and an environment where the athlete's lifestyle, behaviors, and beliefs are discussed • Often attends team training or competition, and travels with team, thus seeing nutrition practice firsthand	• Refers athletes to sports dietitian for assessment and counseling • Where in close access to athletes in daily training environment or travel, implements or monitors team nutrition plan—often acting as the "eyes" or "hands" of the team sports dietitian who has organized plan
Sport psychologist	• Has clinical expertise in diagnosis and management of athletes with eating disorders or disordered eating • Often identifies athletes with food-related stress or poor nutrition practices	• Works within sports medicine team to provide treatment to athletes with eating disorders or disordered eating • Refers athletes to sports dietitian for assessment and counseling • Works with multidisciplinary team to development resources and implement activities related to prevention and early intervention of disordered body image and eating

(Continued)

Table 10.4 *(Continued)*

Professional	Expertise or Opportunities in Sports Nutrition	Roles in Promoting Nutrition in Injury Prevention/Treatment
Sport scientist or exercise physiologist	• Often has expertise in monitoring body physique • Undertakes routine monitoring of physiological, metabolic, and performance status of athletes	• Monitors physique and conditioning, including success of nutrition-related factors in program • Cooperates with sports dietitian to plan and implement activities to alter physique and conditioning • Refers athletes to sports dietitian for assessment and counseling
Coach	• Has day-to-day contact with athlete or team and may observe poor nutritional practice • Has strong influence on many nutritional beliefs and practices of athletes (e.g., supplement use, weight management) • May monitor weight and weight management, although this is a sensitive area between athlete and coach • Is the ultimate observer of performance changes in athletes, identifying situations caused by poor nutrition practice or enhancements potentially caused by positive nutrition interventions	• Supports best nutrition practice by athletes • Encourages use of experts to develop and implement sports nutrition programs, policies, and activities within team or sporting group • Recognizes poor nutrition practice or need for nutrition education, leading to referral to sports dietitian • Works as part of sports medicine or sport science team in management of athletes with complex problems (e.g., eating disorders)
Trainer	• Has contact with athlete or team during training and competition and may observe poor nutritional practice • Is responsible for many nutritional practices or implementation of nutritional plan during training/rehab and competition	• Supports best nutrition practice by athletes • Recognizes poor nutrition practice or need for nutrition education, leading to referral to sports dietitian • During training or competition, implements or monitors team nutrition plan—often acting as the "eyes" or "hands" of the team sports dietitian who has organized plan

Adapted from Burke, L.M. (2007).

Reference

Hespel, P., Op't Eijnde, B., Van Leemputte, M., Ursø, B., Greenhaff, P.L., Labarque, V., Dymarkowski, S., Van Hecke, P. & Richter, E.A. (2001) Oral creatine supplementation facilitates the rehabilitation of disuse atrophy and alters the expression of muscle myogenic factors in humans. *Journal of Physiology*, 15(536), 625–633.

Further readings

Arnold, M. & Barbul, A. (2006) Nutrition and wound healing. *Plastic and Reconstructive Surgery*, 117, 42S–58S.

Burke, L.M. (2007) *Practical Sports Nutrition*. Human Kinetics, Illinois.

Demling, R.H. (2009) Nutrition, anabolism, and the wound healing process: an overview. *Eplasty*, 9, e9.

Glover, E.I. & Phillips, S.M. (2010) Resistance exercise and appropriate nutrition to counteract muscle wasting and promote muscle hypertrophy. *Current Opinion in Clinical Nutrition and Metabolic Care*, 13(6), 630–634.

Nattiv, A., Loucks, A.B., Manore, M.M., Sanborn, C.F., Sundgot-Borgen, J., Warren, M.P. & American College of Sports Medicine (2007) American College of Sports Medicine position stand. The female athlete triad. *Medicine and Science in Sports and Exercise*, 39, 1867–1882.

Stechmiller, J.K. (2010) Understanding the role of nutrition and wound healing. *Nutrition in Clinical Practice*, 25, 61–68.

Tipton, K.D. (2010) Nutrition for acute exercise-induced injuries. *Annals of Nutrition and Metabolism*, 57 (Suppl. 2), 43–53.

Willis, K.S., Peterson, N.J. & Larson-Meyer, D.E. (2008) Should we be concerned about the vitamin D status of athletes? *International Journal of Sport Nutrition and Exercise Metabolism*, 18(2), 204–224.

Appendix: Olympic sports medicine contacts

James Green II[1] and Gayle Olson[2]

[1]MGH Institute of Health Professions, Charlestown, MA, USA
[2]Massachusetts General Hospital, Boston, MA, USA

When traveling internationally with a team, having appropriate contact information regarding sports medicine specialists and operations in the country the team is traveling to would be very useful. This information would be helpful in facilitating planning, logistics and communication, and assuring the best level of care should injury or illness occur when in another country.

While the IOC Directory lists the National Organizing Committees' contact information, no specific information is available regarding sports medicine and key contacts at the National Organizing Committee level in this area. Who to contact concerning the information that is needed by sports medicine specialists traveling with teams or specific questions that they might have or want to discuss prior to traveling would be valuable for all athletes and teams traveling internationally.

In an attempt to develop this information, we contacted each country's National Organizing Committee; based on the information available in the IOC Directory, an email request/letter was sent requesting information that could be collated into a single source within this handbook.

Of the 216 requests that we sent, we received a total of 17 responses. Unfortunately, this was not the response that we had hoped for that would allow us to collate this information on each country in a single source. Due to the lack of full information from the majority of the members of the IOC, we have chosen to list only the main contact information that is available in the IOC Directory.

We continue to believe that having a central source regarding sports medicine resources and personnel at the IOC level or elsewhere would be valuable for teams and the sports medicine specialists who support them, if it could be developed. Such a resource would help assure that the injured athlete receives the best care possible should injury or illness occur during international travel.

Though the information we originally sought is not included in the table, we hope that this table will provide the reader with the ability to contact the National Organizing Committee of the country they may be traveling to in order to attempt to obtain any pretravel information on sports medicine resources available in that country.

Sports Therapy Services, First Edition. Edited by James E. Zachazewski and David J. Magee.
© 2012 International Olympic Committee. Published 2012 by John Wiley & Sons, Ltd.

National Olympic Committees*	Address**
Afghanistan	P.O. Box 1824 GPO, Kabul, Afghanistan
Albania	P.O. Box 63, Sheshi Mustafa K. Ataturk, (ish 21 Dhjetori), Tirane, Albania
Algeria	Case postale 460, Ben Aknoun, Alger 16306, Algeria
American Samoa	P.O. Box 5380, Pago Pago 96799, American Samoa
Andorra	Edf. Principat A 1-2, Av. Tarragona 101, Andorra La Vella, Andorra
Angola	CP 3814, Citadela Desportiva, Luanda, Angola
Antigua and Barbuda	P.O. Box 3115, Redcliffe Street, St John's, Antigua and Barbuda
Argentina	Juncal No 1662, C1062ABV Buenos Aires, Argentina
Armenia	Abovyan Street 9, 0001 Yerevan, Armenia
Aruba	P.O. Box 1175, Complejo Deport. Guillermo Trinidad, Oranjestad, Aruba
Australia	P.O. Box 312, St Leonards, NSW 1590, Australia
Austria	Waldstrasse 14, 2522 Oberwaltersdorf, Austria
Azerbaijan	Olympic Street bl. 5, AZ 370072 Baku, Azerbaijan
Bahamas	P.O. Box SS-6250, Unit 5 Quantum Plaza, Soldier Rd, Nassau N.P., Bahamas
Bahrain	P.O. Box 26406, Manama, Bahrain
Bangladesh	Bhaban, RAJUK Avenue, Outer Stadium, Purana Paltan, Dhaka 1000, Bangladesh
Barbados	Olympic Centre, Garfield Sobers Sports Complex, Wildey, St. Michael BB15094, Barbados
Belarus	Y. Kolasa Street 2, 220050 Minsk, Belarus
Belgium	Avenue de Bouchout 9, 1020 Bruxelles, Belgium
Belize	P.O. Box 384, 1 King Street, Belize City, Belize
Benin	03 BP 2767, Cotonou, Benin
Bermuda	P.O. Box HM 1665, Hamilton HM GX, Bermuda
Bhutan	P.O. Box 939, Thimphu, Bhutan
Bolivia	Casilla postal 4481, Calle México No 1744, La Paz, Bolivia
Bosnia and Herzegovina	Olimpijska dvorana ZETRA, Alipasina bb, 71000 Sarajevo, Bosnia and Herzegovina
Botswana	Private Bag 00180, Gaborone, Botswana
Brazil	Avenida das Americas, 899 Barra da Tijuca, Rio de Janeiro RJ, 22631-000, Brazil
British Virgin Islands	P.O. Box 209, 9, J.R.O Neal Plaza Business, Road Town, Tortola, Virgin Islands, British
Brunei Darussalam	P.O. Box 2008, Bandar Seri Begawan BS8674, Brunei Darussalam
Bulgaria	4, Angel Kanchev Street, 1000 Sofia, Bulgaria
Burkina Faso	01 B.P. 3925, Stade du 4 Août, Porte n° 13, Ouagadougou 01, Burkina Faso
Burundi	B.P. 6247, Avenue du 18 Septembre No 10, Rohero 1, Bujumbura, Burundi
Cambodia	No. 1, Street 276, Beung Keng Kang II, P.O. Box 101, Phnom Penh 12303, Cambodia
Cameroon	P.O. Box 528, Yaoundé, Cameroon
Canada	21 St Clair Avenue East, Suite 900, Toronto ON M4T 1L9, Canada
Cape Verde	P.O. Box 92 A, Rua da UCCLA, Achada de Santo António, Praia, Cape Verde
Cayman Islands	P.O. Box 1786, Grand Cayman KY1-1109, Cayman Islands
Central African Republic	Boîte postale 1541, Rue de Lakouanga, Bangui, Central African Republic
Chad	B.P. 4383, N'djamena Moursal, Chad
Chile	Avenida Ramón Cruz N° 1176, Comuna de Ñuñoa, 2239 Santiago, Chile
Chinese Taipei	Chu-lun St. 20, 104 Taipei, Chinese Taipei
Colombia	Apartado Aéreo 5093, Avenida 68 N° 55-65, Santafé De Bogotá, D.C., Colombia
Comoros	B.P. 1025, Moroni, Comoros
Congo	Boîte postale 1007, Brazzaville, Congo
Cook Islands	P.O. Box 569, Rarotonga, Cook Islands
Costa Rica	P.O. Box 81-2200, Coronado, 1000 San José, Costa Rica
Côte d'Ivoire	08 BP 1212, Abidjan 08, Côte d'Ivoire
Croatia	Trg Kresimira Cosica 11, 10000 Zagreb, Croatia
Cuba	Zona Postal 4, Calle 13 No 601, ESQ. C Vedado, CP 10400 La Habana, Cuba
Cyprus	Olympic House, Olympic House, P.O. Box 23931, 1687 Nicosia, Cyprus
Czech Republic	Benesovská 6, 101 00 Prague 10, Czech Republic
Democratic People's Republic of Korea	P.O. Box 56, Kumsong-dong 2 Kwangbok Street, Mangyongdae District, Pyongyang, Democratic People's Republic of Korea
Democratic Republic of the Congo	Avenue Dima 10, Kinshasa, Democratic Republic of the Congo

National Olympic Committees*	Address**
Denmark	Idraettens Hus, Broendby Stadion 20, 2605 Broendby, Denmark
Djibouti	9, rue de Genève, P.O. Box 1366, Djibouti
Dominica	40 Hillsborough Street, Roseau, Dominica
Dominican Republic	Apartado postal 406, Ave. Pedro Henríquez Ureña 107, Sector la Esperille, Santo Domingo, Dominican Republic
Ecuador	Explanada del Estadio Modelo, Avenida de las Américas, Casilla 09-01-10619, Guayaquil, Ecuador
Egypt	Boîte postale 2055, Rue El Estad El Bahary, Nasr City, Cairo, Egypt
El Salvador	Apartado postal 759, 45 Av. Sur No. 512, Colonia Flor Blanca, San Salvador, El Salvador
Equatorial Guinea	p.a. Ministerio de Educación y Deportes, Apartado postal 847, Malabo, Equatorial Guinea
Eritrea	P.O. Box 7677, Asmara, Eritrea
Estonia	Pirita tee 12, 10127 Tallinn, Estonia
Ethiopia	Axum Building, Ghana Street, P.O. Box 5160, Addis-Abeba, Ethiopia
Federated States of Micronesia	P.O. Box PS 319, Palikir, 96941 Pohnpei Fm, Federated States of Micronesia
Fiji	P.O. Box 1279, Bau Street 17, Suva, Fiji
Finland	Radiokatu 20, 00240 Helsinki, Finland
Former Yugoslav Republic of Macedonia	P.O. Box 914, Bul. Kuzman Josifovski Pitu 17, 1000 Skopje, Macedonia, Ex-Yugoslav Rep. of
France	Maison du Sport Français, 1, avenue Pierre-de-Coubertin, 75640 Paris Cedex 13, France
Gabon	Boîte Postale 802, Libreville, Gabon
Gambia	Bertil Harding Highway, Olympic House, P.O. Box 605, Mile 7, Bakau, Gambia
Georgia	2, Dolidze street, 0102 Tbilisi, Georgia
Germany	Otto-Fleck-Schneise 12, 60528 Frankfurt-Am-Main, Germany
Ghana	P.O. Box 19032, Accra North, Ghana
Great Britain	60 Charlotte Street, London, W1T 2NU, Great Britain
Greece	52, Avenue Dimitrios Vikelas, 152 33 Halandri Athènes, Greece
Grenada	Woolwich Road, P.O. Box 370, St George's, Grenada
Guam	715 Route 8, Maite 96915, Guam
Guatemala	P.O. Box 025368, Miami FL 33102, United States of America
Guinea	Boîte postale 1993, Avenue de la République, Conakry, Guinea
Guinea-Bissau	CP 32, R. Justino Lopes 21 A, Bissau, Guinea-Bissau
Guyana	P.O. Box 10133, Olympic House, 76 High Street, Kingston, Georgetown, Guyana
Haiti	No. 48, Rue Clerveaux, Pétion-Ville, Haiti
Honduras	Complejo Deportivo J. Simón Azcona, Casa Olímpica 'Julio C. Villalta', Apartado postal 3143, Tegucigalpa M.D.C, Honduras
Hong Kong	2/F Olympic House, 1 Stadium Path, So Kon Po, Causeway Bay, Hong Kong, Hong Kong, China
Hungary	Budapest, Magyar Sportok Háza, Istvánmezei út 1-3, 1146, Hungary
Iceland	Engjavegur 6, Sports Center Laugardalur, 104 Reykjavik, Iceland
India	Olympic Bhavan, B-29, Qutab Institutional Area, New Delhi 110016, India
Indonesia	Gedung Direksi Gelora Bung Karno, Jalan Pintu I Senayan, Jakarta 10270, Indonesia
Iraq	P.O. Box 441, Karada, Arasat Street, Baghdad, Iraq
Ireland	Olympic House, Harbour Road, Howth, Dublin, Ireland
Islamic Republic of Iran	North Seoul Ave., Niyayesh Highway, 19956-14336 Tehran, Islamic Republic of Iran
Israel	P.O. Box 53310, 6 Shitrit street, 69482 Tel-Aviv, Israel
Italy	Foro Italico, 00194 Roma, Italy
Jamaica	9 Cunningham Avenue, Kingston 6, Jamaica
Japan	Kishi Memorial Hall, 1-1-1 Jinnan, Shibuya-ku, Tokyo, 150-8050, Japan
Jordan	P.O. Box 19258, Amman 11196, Jordan
Kazakhstan	77, Zhambul street, Almaty, 050000, Kazakhstan
Kenya	P.O. Box 46888, Olympic House, Upper Hill, Kenya Road, Nairobi, 00100, Kenya

National Olympic Committees*	Address**
Kiribati	P.O. Box 238, Bairiki, Tarawa, Kiribati
Korea	Olympic Centre, Oryun-dong Songpa-ku 88, Seoul 138-749, Republic of Korea
Kuwait	IOC NOC Relations Department, Château de Vidy, 1007 Lausanne, Switzerland
Kyrgyzstan	720001 Bishkek, Prospect Chui 207, Kyrgyzstan
Lao People's Democratic Republic	CP 3183, Signy-Centre, Khounbourom Road, Vientiane, Lao People's Democratic Republic
Latvia	Elizabetes Street 49, Riga 1010, Latvia
Lebanon	P.O. Box 23, St Charles Hospital Street, Tony Khoury's Bldg, 1st Floor, Hazmieh Beirut, Lebanon
Lesotho	P.O. Box 756, Kingsway, Maseru 100, Lesotho
Liberia	P.O. Box 6242, 1000 Monrovia 10, Liberia
Libyan Arab Jamahiriya	Omar Al Mukhtar Street, P.O. Box 879, Tripoli, Libyan Arab Jamahiriya
Liechtenstein	Postfach 427, Im Rietacker 4, 9494 Schaan, Liechtenstein
Lithuania	15, Rue Olimpieciu, 09200 Vilnius, Lithuania
Luxembourg	3, route d'Arlon, 8009 Strassen, Luxembourg
Madagascar	Villa Mahatazana, PR II J149, Ambohijatovo Analamahitsy, 101 Antananarivo, Madagascar
Malawi	P.O. Box 867, Along Masauko Chipembere Highway, Sports Council Building, Blantyre, Malawi
Malaysia	Mezzanine Floor, Wisma OCM, Hang Jebat Road, 50150 Kuala Lumpur, Malaysia
Maldives	2nd Floor, Youth and Sports Development Centre, Abadah Ufaa Magu, Male 2005, Maldives
Mali	B.P. 88, Bamako, Mali
Malta	National Swimming Pool Complex, Maria Teresa Spinelli Street, Gzira GZR 1711, Malta
Marshall Islands	P.O. Box 3002, Majuro 96960, Marshall Islands
Mauritania	B.P. 1360, Nouakchott, Mauritania
Mauritius	2nd Floor, Labourdonnais Court, St Georges Street, Port-Louis, Mauritius
Mexico	Apartado postal 36 024, Av. del Conscripto y Anillo Perif., Lomas de Sotelo, 11200 Mexico D.F., Mexico
Monaco	7 avenue des Castelans, Stade Louis II, 98000 Monaco, Monaco
Mongolia	Olympic House, Chinggis Avenue, Ulaanbaatar, 210648, Mongolia
Montenegro	19, Decembra 21, 81000 Podgorica, Republic of Montenegro
Morocco	p.a. Siège des Sports, Boulevard Ibn Sina Aguedal 51, B.P. 134, Rabat, Morocco
Mozambique	Caixa postal 1404, Rua Mateus Sansao Muthemba 397 -431, Maputo, Mozambique
Myanmar (ex Burma until 1989)	Nat. Indoor Stadium (1), Thuwunna, Thingangyun Township, Yangon, Myanmar
Namibia	P.O. Box 21162, Windhoek, Namibia
Nauru	P.O. Box 7, Nauru, Nauru
Nepal	P.O. Box 11455, Satdobato, Lalitpur, Nepal
The Netherlands	P.O. Box 302, Papendallaan 60, 6800 AH Arnhem, The Netherlands
The Netherlands Antilles	P.O. Box 3495, Laufferstrasse z/n, Willemstad, Curacao N.a., The Netherlands Antilles
New Zealand	P.O. Box 643, Wellington 6140, New Zealand
Nicaragua	Residencial Las Palmas, Iglesia Las Palmas, 80 Vrs. al Este, 4981, Managua, Nicaragua
Niger	B.P. 11975, 8000 Niamey, Niger
Nigeria	National Stadium, Surulere, P.O. Box 3156, Marina, Lagos, Nigeria
Norway	Servicebox 1, Ulleval Stadion, 0840 Oslo, Norway
Oman	P.O. Box 2842, 112, Ruwi, Oman
Pakistan	Olympic House, Hameed Nizami Road (Temple Road) 2, Lahore 54000, Pakistan
Palau	P.O. Box 155, 96940 Koror, Palau
Palestine	P.O. Box 469, 9727 Gaza, Palestine
Panama	Avenida Ricardo J. Alfaro, Edificio Fenacota, 4° Piso, Oficina 401, Loceria, Panama City, Panama
Papua New Guinea	P.O. Box 467, Boroko 111 NCD, Papua New Guinea
Paraguay	Casilla Postal 1420, Medallistas Olímpicos 1, Asuncion, Paraguay

National Olympic Committees*

Address**

People's Republic of China	Tiyuguan Road 2, Beijing 100763, République populaire de Chine
Peru	Cesar Vallejo No 290, Lima 14, Peru
Philippines	PSC-Building A, Philsports Complex, Meralco Avenue, 1603 Pasig City, Philippines
Poland	Wybrzeze Gdynskie 4, 01-531 Varsovie, Poland
Portugal	Travessa da Memoria no. 36, 1300-403 Lisboa, Portugal
Puerto Rico	Casa Olímpica, Apartado 9020008, San Juan 00902-0008, Puerto Rico
Qatar	P.O. Box 7494, Olympic Building, Doha, Qatar
Republic of Moldova	Rue Puskin 11, MD-2012 Chisinau, Republic of Moldova
Romania	155 Calea Victoriei, BI. D1, Tronson 5, 3rd floor, Sector 1, 10073 Bucarest, Romania
Russian Federation	Luzhnetskaya Nab. 8, Moscow, 119992, Russian Federation
Rwanda	B.P. 2684, Stade National Amahoro de Remera, Kigali, Rwanda
Saint Kitts and Nevis	P.O. Box 953, Olympic House, No. 18 Taylors Range, Basseterre, Saint Kitts and Nevis
Saint Lucia	P.O. Box CP 6023, Barnard Hill, Castries, Saint Lucia
Saint Vincent and the Grenadines	P.O. Box 1644, Kingstown, St Vincent and the Grenadines
Samoa (until 1996 Western Samoa)	P.O. Box 1301, Apia, Samoa
San Marino	Via Rancaglia 30, 47899 Serravalle, San Marino
Sao Tome and Principe	Caixa postal 630, Palacio dos Pioneiros, Salas 9 e 10, Quinta de Santo Antonio, Sao Tomé, Sao Tome and Principe
Saudi Arabia	P.O. Box 6040, Prince Faisal Fahd Olympic Complex, Riyadh 11442, Saudi Arabia
Senegal	Boîte postale 356, Dakar, Senegal
Serbia	Generala Vasica 5, 11040 Belgrade, Serbia
Seychelles	P.O. Box 584, Victoria Mahe, Seychelles
Sierra Leone	Howe Street 25, P.M. Bag 639, Freetown, Sierra Leone
Singapore	Singapore Sports Council Building, West Wing--2nd Storey, 230 Stadium Boulevard, Singapore 397799, Singapore
Slovakia	Kukucinova 26, 838 08 Bratislava, Slovakia
Slovenia	Celovska 25, 1000 Ljubljana, Slovenia
Solomon Islands	NSC Building, Kukum High Wy, P.O. Box 532, Honiara, Solomon Islands
Somalia	DHL Mogadishu, Mogadishu, Somalia
South Africa	P.O. Box 1355, Houghton, Johannesburg 2041, South Africa
Spain	Calle Arequipa 13, Gran Via de Hortaleza, 28043 Madrid, Spain
Sri Lanka	No. 100/9 F, Independence Avenue, Colombo 7, Sri Lanka
Sudan	P.O. Box 1938, Africa Street, Khartoum, Sudan
Suriname	P.O. Box 3043, Letitia Vriesdalan Olympic Center, Paramaribo, Suriname
Swaziland	P.O. Box 835, Mbabane, H100, Swaziland
Sweden	Sofiatornet Olympiastadion, 114 33 Stockholm, Sweden
Switzerland	Postfach 606, 3000 Berne 22, Switzerland
Syrian Arab Republic	P.O. Box 3375, Avenue Baramke, Damascus, Syrian Arab Republic
Tadjikistan	P.O. Box 2, Aini Street 24, 734025 Dushanbe, Tajikistan
Thailand	Banampawan Sriayudhaya Road 226, Dusit Bangkok 10300, Thailand
Timor-Leste	P.O. Box 137, Avenida de Lisboa, Dili, Democratic Republic of Timor-Leste
Togo	Boîte postale 1320, Angle Av. Duisburg-Rue des Nîmes, Lomé, Togo
Tonga	P.O. Box 1278, Vaha'akolo Road, Haveluloto, Nuku'alofa, Tonga
Trinidad and Tobago	P.O. Box 529, 121 Abercromby St, Port of Spain, Trinidad and Tobago
Tunisia	Centre Cult. & Sp. de la Jeunesse, Av. Othman Ibn Afane El Menzah VI, 1004 Tunis, Tunisia
Turkey	Olimpiyatevi/Olympic House, Kisim Sonu 4, 34158 Atakoy-Istanbul, Turkey
Turkmenistan	76, Garashsyzlyk Street, 744013 Ashgabat, Turkmenistan
Tuvalu	Private Mail Bag, Funafuti, Tuvalu
Uganda	Plot 2-10 Hesketh Bell Road, Lugogo Sports Complex, P.O. Box 2610, Kampala, Uganda
Ukraine	Esplanadna St. 42, 01601 Kiev, Ukraine

National Olympic Committees*

	Address**
United Arab Emirates	P.O. Box 4350, Block B Office No. 701, Dubai, United Arab Emirates
United Republic of Tanzania	P.O. Box 2182, National Housing Cooperation, 3rd Floor no. 2, Mwinyijuma Road, Mwananyamala, Dar-Es-Salaam, United Republic of Tanzania
United States of America	1 Olympic Plaza, Colorado Springs CO 80909, United States of America
Uruguay	Casilla postal 161, Calle Canelones 1044, Montevideo, 11100, Uruguay
Uzbekistan	Almazar Street 15/1, 100003 Tashkent, Uzbekistan
Vanuatu	P.O. Box 284, Port Vila, Vanuatu
Venezuela	Urb. El Paraiso, Avenida Estadio, Edificio Comité Olímpico Venezolano, Caracas 1020, Venezuela
Vietnam	Tran Phu Street 36, Badinh District, Hanoi, Vietnam
Virgin Islands	P.O. Box 366, Frederiksted, Sainte-Croix 00841, Virgin Islands, USA
Yemen	Althawrah Sports City Complex, P.O. Box 2701, Sana'a, Yemen
Zambia	P.O. Box 36119, 10101 Lusaka, Zambia
Zimbabwe	3 Aintree Circle, Belvedere, Harare, Zimbabwe

*http://www.olympic.org/ioc-governance-national-olympic-committees?tab=0
**http://www.olympic.org/national-olympic-committees

Index

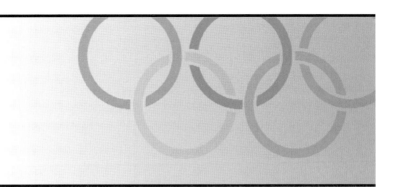

Note: Page numbers with italicized *f*'s and *t*'s refer to figures and tables, respectively.

Sports Therapy Services, First Edition. Edited by James E. Zachazewski and David J. Magee.
© 2012 International Olympic Committee. Published 2012 by John Wiley & Sons, Ltd.